N02638

Colorectal Cancer

Colorectal cancer is the second most common cause of cancer death in the developed world. The last five years have seen dramatic improvements in the multidisciplinary management of this malignancy. In this book, experts at the forefront of these advances contribute their knowledge and experience on the major advances that have occurred in diagnosis, staging, preoperative and adjuvant therapy, surgery and follow-up assessment of patients with this disease. Imaging underpins all aspects of the clinical management of colorectal cancer and has been shown to play a critical role in improving outcomes for patients.

Gina Brown

Contemporary Issues in Cancer Imaging

A Multidisciplinary Approach

Series Editors

Rodney H. Reznek
Cancer Imaging, St. Bartholomew's Hospital, London

Janet E. Husband
Diagnostic Radiology, Royal Marsden Hospital, Surrey

Current titles in the series

Cancer of the Ovary
Lung Cancer

Forthcoming titles in the series

Carcinoma of the Kidney
Carcinoma of the Esophagus
Carcinoma of the Bladder
Prostate Cancer
Squamous Cell Cancer of the Neck
Pancreatic Cancer
Interventional Radiological Treatment of Liver Tumours

Colorectal Cancer

Edited by

Gina Brown

Series Editors

Rodney H. Reznek

Janet E. Husband

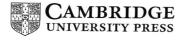

CAMBRIDGE
UNIVERSITY PRESS

CAMBRIDGE UNIVERSITY PRESS
Cambridge, New York, Melbourne, Madrid, Cape Town, Singapore, São Paulo

Cambridge University Press
The Edinburgh Building, Cambridge CB2 8RU, UK

Published in the United States of America by Cambridge University Press, New York

www.cambridge.org
Information on this title: www.cambridge.org/9780521692915

© Cambridge University Press 2007

This publication is in copyright. Subject to statutory exception
and to the provisions of relevant collective licensing agreements,
no reproduction of any part may take place without
the written permission of Cambridge University Press.

First published 2007

Printed in the United Kingdom at the University Press, Cambridge

A catalog record for this publication is available from the British Library

Library of Congress Cataloging in Publication Data
Colorectal cancer / edited by Gina Brown.
    p.   cm. – (Contemporary issues in cancer imaging)
Includes bibliographical references.
ISBN 978-0-521-69291-5 (hardback)
1. Colon (Anatomy) – Cancer.   2. Rectum – Cancer.   I. Brown, Gina.   II. Title.   III. Series.
[DNLM: 1. Colorectal Neoplasms – diagnosis.   2. Colorectal Neoplasms.   3. Diagnostic Imaging – methods.
WI 529 C7189 2007]
RC280.C6C6626   2007
616.99′4347–dc22   2007022029

ISBN 978-0-521-69291-5 hardback

Cambridge University Press has no responsibility for
the persistence or accuracy of URLs for external or
third-party internet websites referred to in this publication,
and does not guarantee that any content on such
websites is, or will remain, accurate or appropriate.

Every effort has been made in preparing this publication to provide accurate and up-to-date information which is
in accord with accepted standards and practice at the time of publication. Although case histories are drawn from
actual cases, every effort has been made to disguise the identities of the individuals involved. Nevertheless, the
authors, editors and publishers can make no warranties that the information contained herein is totally free from
error, not least because clinical standards are constantly changing through research and regulation. The authors,
editors and publishers therefore disclaim all liability for direct or consequential damages resulting from the use of
material contained in this publication. Readers are strongly advised to pay careful attention to information
provided by the manufacturer of any drugs or equipment that they plan to use.

Contents

Contributors

Mr. Anthony Antoniou, BSC MBBCHIR FRCS
The Royal Marsden Hospital
Fulham Road
London SW3 6JJ

Dr. Gina Brown, MBBS MD MRCP FRCR
Consultant Radiologist and Honorary Senior
  Lecturer
Royal Marsden Hospital
Downs Road
Sutton
Surrey SM2 5PT

Ms. Sarah Burton, BMBS MS FRCS
Consultant Colorectal Surgeon
Frimley Park Hospital
Portsmouth Road
Frimley

Dr. Peter Chowdhury, MB BCH FRCR
Consultant Radiologist
Swansea NHS Trust
Swansea
UK

Dr. Yu Jo Chua, MBBS
Department of Medicine
Royal Marsden Hospital
Downs Road
Sutton
Surrey SM2 5PT
UK

Prof. David Cunningham, MD FRCP
Department of Medicine
Royal Marsden Hospital
Downs Road
Sutton
Surrey SM2 5PT
UK

Mr. Ian R. Daniels, FRCS
Consultant Surgeon
Royal Devon & Exeter Hospital
Barrack Road
Exeter
Devon EX2 5DW

Prof. Lord Ara Darzi, FRENG KBE FMEDSCI
Paul Hamlyn Chair of Surgery
Professor of Surgery
Division of Surgery
Institute of Cancer Research
Royal Marsden Hospital
Fulham Road
London SW3 3JJ

Dr. Rhodri Davies, MB BCH MD FRCP
Consultant Gastroenterologist
Caerphilly Miners' Hospital
Caerphilly
UK

Ms. Sarah E. Fisher, RGN
RGN Pelican Research Nurse
Pelican Cancer Foundation
North Hampshire Hospital
Aldermaston Road
Basingstoke
Hampshire RG24 9NA

Prof. Steve Halligan, MBBS MD FRCP FRCR
Professor of Gastrointestinal Radiology
Department of Specialist Radiology
Level 2 Podium
University College Hospital
235 Euston Road
London NW1 2BU

Prof. Richard J. Heald, OBE MCHIR FRCS
Surgical Director
Pelican Cancer Foundation
North Hampshire Hospital
Aldermaston Road
Basingstoke
Hampshire RG24 9NA

Dr. Brian D. P. O'Neill, MB MRCPI FFRRCSI
Clinical Research Fellow in GI Clinical Oncology
Royal Marsden Hospital
Sutton
Surrey SM2 5PT
UK

Prof. Philip Quirke, BM PHD FRCPATH
Gastrointestinal Cancer Research Group
Pathology and Tumour Biology
Yorkshire Cancer Research and Liz Dawn
Translational Science Centre
Leeds Institute of Molecular Medicine
Wellcome Trust Brenner Building
St James University Hospital
Becket Street
Leeds LS9 7TF
UK

Dr. Ashley Roberts, MB BCH MD MRCP FRCR
Consultant Radiologist
University Hospital of Wales
Cardiff CF14 4XW
UK

Dr. Naureen Starling, BSC MRCP
Specialist Registrar
Royal Marsden Hospital
Sutton
Surrey SM2 5PT
UK

Dr. Diana M. Tait, MD FRCP FRCR
Department of Clinical Oncology
Royal Marsden Hospital
Sutton
Surrey SM2 5PT
UK

Series foreword

Imaging has become pivotal in all aspects of the management of patients with cancer. At the same time, it is acknowledged that optimal patient care is best achieved by a multidisciplinary team approach. The explosion of technological developments in imaging over the past years has meant that all members of the multidisciplinary team should understand the potential applications, limitations, and advantages of all the evolving and exciting imaging techniques. Equally, to understand the significance of the imaging findings and to contribute actively to management decisions and the development of new clinical applications for imaging, it is critical that the radiologist should have sufficient background knowledge of different tumors. Thus, the radiologist should understand the pathology, the clinical background, the therapeutic options, and prognostic indicators of malignancy.

Contemporary Issues in Cancer Imaging: A Multidisciplinary Approach aims to meet the growing requirement for radiologists to have a detailed knowledge of the individual tumors in which they are involved in making management decisions. A series of single subject issues, each of which will be dedicated to a single tumor site, edited by recognized expert guest editors, will include contributions from basic scientists, pathologists, surgeons, oncologists, radiologists, and others.

While the series is written predominantly for the radiologist, it is hoped that individual issues will contain sufficient varied information so as to be of interest to all medical disciplines and to other health professionals managing patients with cancer. As with imaging, advances have occurred in all these disciplines related to cancer management and it is our fervent hope that this series, bringing together expertise from such a range of related specialties, will not only promote the understanding and rational application of modern imaging but will also help to achieve the ultimate goal of improving outcomes for patients with cancer.

Rodney H. Reznek
London

Janet E. Husband
London

Acknowledgements

We would like to express our gratitude to all our contributors to this colorectal edition, who have so generously given up their time to make such excellent contributions to this project. Their contributions and specialist expertise have made this a unique, multi-disciplinary, state-of-the-art summary of the optimum management of this disease.

Finally we would like to acknowledge the many hours of dedication and patience that Ms Barbara Mason has put into this project in collating material, helping with the editorial amendments and the production of the images.

The clinical presentation of colorectal cancer

Sarah E. Fisher and Ian R. Daniels

Introduction

Colorectal cancer is the second commonest cancer arising in the United Kingdom. In this chapter, we will discuss the etiology involving genetic and environmental factors, the presenting features of the disease, the clinical findings and the referral process.

Incidence and mortality

In 1996, colorectal cancer (CRC) accounted for over 15 000 deaths (68% colon, 32% rectal) and, by the turn of the millennium, there had been 33 173 new cases of CRC diagnosed in the UK in the previous 12 months. Stratified by sex, the incidence per 100 000 of the population (all ages) is 53.5–57.1 cases for men and 36.7–37.5 cases for women. The average age of diagnosis is in the 60–65 year group. The incidence by age stratification is 4 cases/100 000 for people under the age of 50; 100 cases/100 000 for those aged 50–69; and 300 cases/100 000 for those over the age of 70 [1,2]. In Australia, the UK, and the United States, it is the commonest cancer in women after breast (age standardization 22–33 cases/100 000) and in men after prostate and lung cancer (age standardized incidence 31–47 cases/100 000) [3]. Overall, it accounts for approximately 10% of all cancer deaths (Table 1.1) [1].

Survival rates for colorectal cancer have improved in recent years. Between the 1970s and 1990s, 5-year survival for colon cancer in men improved from 22% to 42% and rectal cancer rates improved from 25% to 39%. For colon cancer in women, 5-year survival increased from 23% to 40% and rectal cancer from 27% to 43%. Indeed, we are now seeing series reported with a higher survival rate for

Table 1.1   The incidence and deaths from colorectal cancer worldwide

	Incidence	Incidence ASR	Deaths	Deaths ASR
World				
Men	498 754	19.11	254 816	9.78
Women	445 963		237 595	7.58
UK				
Men	17 249	35.37	9 341	18.73
Women	15 924	25.28	9 047	13.76

Incidence and age-standardized ratio (ASR) expressed per 100 000 people [1].

rectal than colon cancer [4]. This probably relates to earlier detection of the disease and to the introduction of multidisciplinary team management of the disease. But, with an increasing elderly population in the UK, the incidence of CRC will rise and this will add to the burden on NHS cancer services.

Risk factors

A number of environmental and genetic risk factors have been identified for CRC. These include
- Age
- Nutrition
- Low physical activity
- Inflammatory bowel disease
- Genetic factors

It is estimated that about 80% of all cases of CRC are caused by diet alone [5]. Colorectal cancer is more common in Westernized countries than in Asia or Africa – the increased consumption of dietary fiber in the form of fruit, vegetables and cereals has been proposed as a protective factor. A high-fiber diet increases fecal bulk and decreases transit time. The issue of dietary fiber intake and the relationship to the risk of CRC were highlighted by the observations of Dennis Burkitt in the 1970s and 1980s, but these observations have recently been disputed [6]. There is evidence that a diet rich in red or processed meat may increase the risk [7]. The EPIC (European Prospective Investigation into Cancer and Nutrition) Study identified an increased risk with total consumption of meat [8]. The evidence for the effect of dietary fat is not consistent [9]. Folate has been shown to have a protective effect in a number of prospective cohort studies, and a number of randomized control trials have demonstrated a decreased risk of recurrent adenomas with calcium supplements. Selenium may also have an anti-carcinogenic effect. Whilst alcohol increases the risk for CRC, the evidence for tobacco is inconclusive.

Epidemiological studies have highlighted that men who are physically active are at decreased risk of developing CRC [10]. There is no consistent link between CRC and obesity but there is an association between obesity and the development of adenomas.

Patients with inflammatory bowel disease, both ulcerative colitis and Crohn's colitis, have a higher risk of developing CRC than the general population. In ulcerative colitis, the cumulative risk is reported as 2% at 10 years, 8% at 20 years and 18% by 30 years [11]. The incidence for Crohn's colitis is reported to be higher. Individuals who develop adenomatous polyps are also at increased risk of developing CRC.

There are a number of protective factors, including a lower incidence in patients taking aspirin. Hormone replacement therapy is also associated with a relative risk reduction. Cyclo-oxygenase-2 (COX-2) inhibitors and the statins have also been shown in population-based studies to provide some protection.

Genetics

Whilst environmental factors probably act as a catalyst in genetically susceptible individuals, there are a number of hereditary factors that increase the likelihood of the development of CRC. When assessing a patient, the question of family history of CRC is often raised, and indeed many patients will have an affected relative, either first-degree (parent or direct sibling) or second-degree (grandparent, aunts, and uncles). However, for a patient presenting to the surgical outpatient clinic, those with a single relative diagnosed over the age of 60 have the same risk as the general population. Indeed, about 25% of patients with CRC have a positive family history. However, heritable factors account for 35% of the risk of developing CRC [12]. These heritable factors can be considered in two groups:

1. High-penetration autosomal dominant syndromes – familial adenomatous polyposis (FAP and variants) and hereditary non-polyposis colorectal cancer (HNPCC), which represent 2%–5% of all colorectal cancers and is associated with an 80% lifetime risk. In FAP families, direct mutation analysis will give positive results in 80% of families. In FAP, the mutation involves a tumor-suppressor gene (APC gene) on loci 5q that is inherited in an autosomal

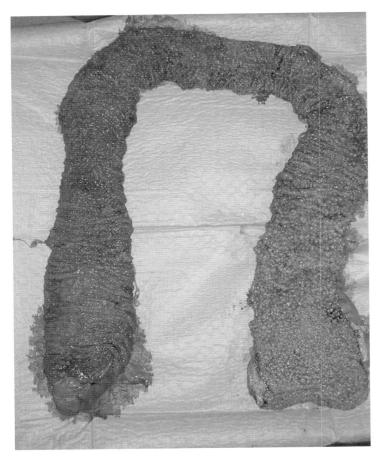

Figure 1.1 A proctocolectomy specimen removed from a patient with polyposis and no previous family history of the condition. The images show the 'carpet' of polyps extending around the entire colon from the anorectal junction to the ileocecal valve. The enlarged view of the rectum reveals the typical appearance of the multiple adenomata.

dominant pattern. The disease is characterized by the development of hundreds to thousands of adenomatous polyps. Depending upon the penetrance, patients may have a few polyps or an entire carpet involving the colon and rectum (Figure 1.1). Variants of the condition include Gardener's syndrome and Turcot's syndrome. In HNPCC, five different genes have been associated with the condition, making direct mutation analysis a more difficult problem. The majority of people have a germ-line mutation in a DNA mis-match repair gene. This microsatellite instability, which may be found at multiple loci, including the 2p and 2q regions, is associated with increased genetic instability. Microsatellites are 50 000–100 000 di-nucleotide (e.g., CACACACA, etc.), tri-nucleotide (GTGCTGCTG, etc.), and tetra-nucleotide repeats that code for DNA repair proteins. Those genes that contain mutations cannot perform this repair function, DNA instability results and a malignancy may develop.

2. Familial clustering is likely to have a multifactorial mode of inheritance. Several genes are likely to be involved, some may predispose to adenomatous polyp formation [13,14]. The mode of inheritance is autosomal dominant but with a low penetrance [15]. The key determinants of risk are the youngest age of onset of CRC and the number of first-degree relatives involved.

Overall, any individual with two affected first-degree relatives aged less than 75 years at diagnosis has over twice the lifetime risk of CRC as compared to the general population. There are no national guidelines for surveillance in this cohort although it is known that these family members develop polyps more frequently than the general population, as has been demonstrated in a population-based screening trial [16]. Polypectomy does lead to a substantial reduction in cancer incidence in this group [17]. Surveillance is usually offered on a 5-yearly basis [18,19,20].

Pathogenesis

The development from a single cellular event to a metastatic tumor occurs in a stepwise progression from normal mucosa to adenoma to invasive carcinoma. The development of a malignancy within the colon is well characterized through the adenoma–carcinoma sequence [21]. The majority of carcinomas develop from benign, pre-neoplastic lesions – adenomatous polyps, following the accumulation of changes that occur within the cells of the lining of the bowel. Although we know the genetic sequence of events within this process, the etiology is multifactorial, involving genetic susceptibility, environmental factors and somatic changes during the initiation and progression of this process [22].

The genetic model for the progression of development of the neoplasm can be represented in a stepwise series of genomic events involving alterations in several oncogenes (K-ras) and tumor-suppressor genes (APC, DCC/DPC4, P53), DNA repair genes (*h*MLH1 and *h*MSH2), cell adhesion molecules (epCam), angiogenic factors (VEGF), as well as epigenetic changes (DNA methylation) and microsatellite instability (Figure 1.2).

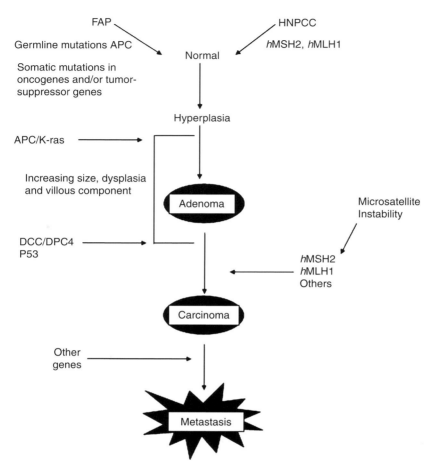

Figure 1.2 Alterations in several oncogenes and tumor-suppressor genes according to the two major mechanisms of genomic instability: microsatellite instability and chromosomal instability.

Symptoms of colorectal cancer

The classic symptoms of large bowel obstruction – abdominal colic, absolute constipation, abdominal distension and vomiting – are now rarely seen in modern colorectal practice. With the increasing influence of health awareness, the population has become more "bowel aware." However, the symptoms of colorectal cancer do not indicate a clear diagnosis as there is considerable similarity with more common colorectal complaints such as irritable bowel syndrome (IBS), inflammatory bowel disease (IBD), diverticulosis and its complications, and proctological conditions such as hemorrhoids. Recent UK data reports a delay of 10 months between onset of symptoms and treatment of CRC, with a median patient delay of 3 months, usually because the patient does not think the symptoms are serious [22]. Much of the work on symptom presentation and delay of treatment was assessed through the Wessex Cancer Audit and the Wales–Trent Audit performed in the 1980s and 1990s [22]. The audits identified that 65% of the delay in patients having elective surgery occurred before referral to hospital, 15% waiting for an outpatient appointment and 20% during the diagnostic process [22]. The figures for proximal bowel cancer (cecum to splenic flexure) were 35% before GP referral, 19% waiting for outpatient appointment and 46% owing to hospital delay in diagnosis.

There was a significant delay in the 15% of patients referred to the physicians, compared to the 85% of patients with suspected CRC referred to the surgical team. In the Wales–Trent Audit this was similar, even when those presenting with anemia were excluded. Therefore, the time to referral, diagnosis and treatment has not changed over the last 20 years [22,23].

Clinical history

Colorectal cancer proximal to the splenic flexure does not usually present with symptoms of bowel cancer. Proximal disease referrals are usually due to the identification of an iron deficiency anemia (microcytic, hypochromic), an abdominal mass, or as an emergency presentation with signs and symptoms of intestinal obstruction [24,25,26]. However, for left colon and rectal cancer, the presentation is usually with rectal bleeding and a change in bowel habit, which is usually an increased frequency of defecation and/or looser stools [27]. Rectal bleeding occurs without anal symptoms in over 60% of patients [27,28]. In very low rectal cancer, the symptom of tenesmus – the feeling of incomplete evacuation – may occur, and anal pain usually indicates that invasion of the anal sphincter has occurred.

Clinical examination

If you don't put your finger in it, you'll put your foot in it.

The old surgical adage, beloved by consultant surgeons and emphasized to junior doctors, does continue to have clinical value. A palpable rectal mass is present in 40%–80% of patients with rectal cancer, and 82% of palpable rectal cancers may be assessed by GPs [29,30,31]. Despite the advances in diagnostic technology, there is much that can be gained by the clinical examination of the patient. In the outpatient setting, a general physical examination of the patient and a digital rectal examination, together with examination using a rigid sigmoidoscope and proctoscope, allow accurate clinical assessment. If a rectal cancer is identified, bi-manual examination of female patients gives the surgeon further information, although magnetic resonance imaging (MRI) assessment may be more accurate for treatment planning.

Having identified a CRC, particularly if it is detected by sigmoidoscopy, it is important that the entire colon is visualized to exclude synchronous lesions, which are reported to occur in 4%–5% [31,32]. The recognition of adenomatous polyps away from the area of resection may lead to a change in the operative strategy. Whilst a barium enema may act as a good investigation to assess proximal bowel, particularly in the presence of a tumor impassable to endoscopic examination, the ideal modality to assess the proximal colon is colonoscopy. However, one of the disadvantages of colonoscopy is the inability to accurately localize the position of the tumor within the colon when planning surgery. A particular area of difficulty is the "malignant polyp" – tattooing of the colon allows the surgeon to accurately identify the area for resection during the operation.

Prior to treatment planning, an accurate clinical and radiological assessment of the patient is performed to stage local disease and to exclude distant disease. The current best practice is local staging by endoscopic assessment of the tumor, with MRI assessment of a rectal cancer, together with a CT scan of the chest, abdomen and pelvis to exclude distant disease. Preoperative investigations including a full blood count and biochemical profile are also important. Serum CEA (carcino-embryonic antigen) is of value only if the level is raised. However, long-term follow-up with a serum CEA is probably of little value as a screening tool for the detection of recurrence in colorectal cancers.

Referral to the multidisciplinary team process

The Calman-Hine Policy Framework for Commissioning Cancer Services first highlighted the need to deliver improved and co-ordinated cancer services with the need for a cancer network infrastructure [33]. The report aimed: "to create a network of care in England and Wales, which will enable a patient, wherever he or she lives to be sure that the treatment and care received is of a uniformly high standard."

Reviewing the published medical literature in the late 1980s and early 1990s, supplemented by registry studies, revealed that there could be significant improvements in survival as a result of specialist care for a number of cancers including colorectal cancer [34,35]. With these developments in mind, the NHS

Cancer Plan was introduced in 2000 to improve the diagnosis and treatment for patients of the five most common cancers [36]. The evidence for this concluded that

1. Patients treated by specialists or specialist units have improved outcomes or process of care [37]
2. Patients treated by surgeons or units with higher patient volumes have improved outcomes or process of care [38]

The establishment of multidisciplinary team (MDT) working with regular meetings to discuss patients and co-ordinate care is seen as a central element for cancer care. The MDT is defined as "a group of different health care disciplines, which meets together at a given time (whether physically in one place or by video or teleconferencing) to discuss a given patient and who are able to contribute independently to the diagnosis and treatment decisions about the patients" [22].

Having set the standards for the management of patients in the hospital setting, the next task was to attempt to improve the referral pattern of patients to hospital and improve on the access to diagnostic services. This led to the "fast-track referral" or "two-week-wait" system (Figures 1.3 and 1.4).

Higher-risk criteria have been identified to allow primary care practitioners to direct patients through a fast-track or two-week-wait referral and these should

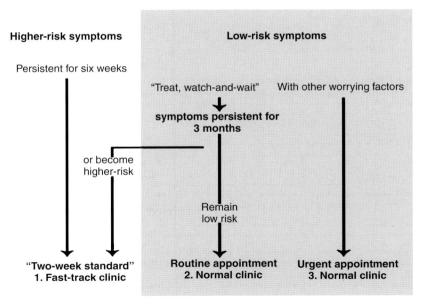

Figure 1.3 **The guidelines for referral of patients with suspected colorectal cancer based upon clinical history and examination by the general practitioner.**

REVIEW DATE: JUNE 2003
SUSPECTED CANCER REFERRAL PROFORMA
COLORECTAL
☒ FAXBACK NUMBER: 0151 706 5655

The Royal Liverpool and **NHS**
Broadgreen University Hospitals
NHS Trust

PATIENT DETAILS		GP DETAILS
NAME:		NAME:
ADDRESS:		ADDRESS:
POSTCODE:	TEL:	
DOB: / /	NHS NO:	FAX NO:
INTERPRETER: YES / NO	LANGUAGE:	DATE OF REFERRAL:

CLINICAL INFORMATION

Please tick the relevant boxes.
OVER 60 YEARS ONLY:

Rectal bleeding persistently **WITHOUT** anal symptoms:
(Anal symptoms include soreness, discomfort, itching, lumps, and prolapse as well as pain)   ☐

Change of bowel habit to looser stools and/or increased frequency of defecation, persistent for 6 weeks **WITHOUT** rectal bleeding   ☐

ALL AGES:

Rectal bleeding **WITH** persistent change in bowel habit to looser stools and/or increased frequency of defecation persistent for 6 weeks   ☐

A definite palpable right-sided abdominal mass with or without abdominal pain.   ☐

A definite palpable rectal (not pelvic) mass   ☐

Iron Deficiency anemia WITHOUT an obvious cause (Hb<11g/dl in men Or <10g/dl in post menopausal women). **Hb: MCV:**   ☐

Tick if patient is fit for Phosphate enema at home prior to Flexible Sigmoidoscopy   ☐

Recent Investigations **(please include all bowel investigations ordered):**
_____
_____
_____

Patients past medical history:
_____
_____
_____

Recent heart attack: Y / N   Date: Angina: Y / N   Stroke: Y / N

Current medication: Warfarin Y / N _____
_____
_____

Further comments:
_____

If you are unsure whether this is the most appropriate method of referral for your patient please contact the colorectal nurse/TWR co-ordinator on 0151 706 3453 (or bleep 261)

Doctors Signature: Date:

Figure 1.4   An example of a referral proforma used.

consist of 80%–90% of all colorectal cancers presenting to surgical outpatients. These criteria are:

- Rectal bleeding with a change in bowel habit to increased frequency of defecation and/or looser stools and persistent for at least 6 weeks – all ages
- Rectal bleeding persistent without anal symptoms – age > 60 years
- Change in bowel habit to increased frequency of defecation and/or looser stools persistent for at least 6 weeks – age > 60 years
- Patients with an easily palpable right iliac fossa mass – all ages
- Patients with an easily palpable intraluminal rectal mass – all ages
- Patients with an unexplained iron deficiency anemia

    Hb < 11 g/dl in men   All ages
    Hb < 10 g/dl in women   Postmenopausal

However, there are also "low-risk symptoms" as it must be appreciated that the risk of colorectal cancer is never zero, as patients may have a cancer and be symptomatic from functional bowel disease or hemorrhoids, etc. This means that all low-risk patients with persistent symptoms who do not respond to treatment or have recurring symptoms should be investigated through a routine outpatient clinic. These criteria include:

- Rectal bleeding with anal symptoms
- Rectal bleeding with an obvious external visible case such as prolapsed piles, rectal prolapse and anal fissure
- Transient changes in bowel habit for < 6 weeks, particularly to a decreased frequency of defecation with straining and harder stools
- Abdominal pain not associated with other high-risk symptoms, iron deficiency anemia, a palpable abdominal or rectal mass, or clearly caused by intestinal obstruction.

Despite the introduction of these guidelines and referral proformas, a considerable number of colorectal cancers present outside of this pattern and the debate as to the effectiveness of the "two-week wait" continue. Against this though must be balanced the treatment targets set up by the Department of Health that give clear guidance as to the maximum length of wait between stages in the multidisciplinary care process.

Screening

As CRC has a high incidence but a relatively long period between the development from adenoma to malignancy and, also results in both high human and financial costs, research into screening for colorectal cancer to detect the disease earlier and improve outcome was undertaken. A number of trials were conducted including fecal occult blood testing (FOB), flexible sigmoidoscopy, and colonoscopy. Four large randomized controlled trials (RCTs) and two large non-RCTs have addressed the effectiveness of FOB testing. The combined evidence from RCTs of hemoccult screening suggests that screening reduces mortality from CRC. The point estimate is 16%, but may range from 7% to 23% [3]. The influence of screening will be further explored in a later chapter.

Conclusion

The incidence of colorectal cancer in the Western world is rising. However, whilst the genetic process underlying the disease is now recognized, as yet this has had little effect on preventing or improving treatment. Improved health awareness through patient education may make a difference, but the biggest improvement will come with screening.

REFERENCES

1. GLOBOCAN (2000). Cancer incidence, mortality and prevalence worldwide. International Agency for Research on Cancer European Network of Cancer Registries (IARC CancerBase No 5) www.dep.iarc.fr.
2. Office of National Statistics (ONS). Monitor. Stationary Office 1997.
3. Towler B., Irwig L., Glasziou P., Weller D., and Kewenter J. A systematic review of the effects of screening for colorectal cancer using the faecal occult blood test, Hemoccult. *BMJ*, **317** (1998), 559–65.
4. Birgisson H., Talback M., Gunnarsson U., Pahlman L., and Glimelius B. Improved survival in cancer of the colon and rectum in Sweden. *EJSO*, **31**(2005), 845–53.
5. Cummings J. H. and Bingham S. A. Diet and the prevention of cancer. *BMJ*, **317** (1998), 1636–40.
6. Bingham S. A., Day N. E., Luben R., *et al.* European Prospective Investigation into Cancer and Nutrition (EPIC). Dietary fibre in food and protection against colorectal cancer in the European Prospective Investigation into Cancer and Nutrition (EPIC): an observational study. *Lancet*, **361** (2003), 1496–501.
7. Linseisen J., Kesse E., Slimani N., *et al.* EPIC Working Group on Dietary Pattern, Subgroup Meat. Meat consumption in Europe: results from the EPIC study. *IARC Sci Publ*, **156** (2002), 211–12.
8. Platz E. A., Giovannucci E., Rimm E. B., *et al.* Dietary fiber and distal colorectal adenoma in men. *Cancer Epidemiol Biomarkers Prev*, **6** (1997), 661–70.

9. Mai V., Flood A., Peters U., *et al.* Dietary fibre and risk of colorectal cancer in the Breast Cancer Detection Demonstration Project (BCDDP) follow-up cohort. *IJE*, **33** (2003), 234–8.

10. Giovannucci E. and Willett W. C. Dietary factors and risk of colon cancer. *Ann Med*, **26** (1994), 443–52.

11. Eaden J. A., Abrams K. R., and Mayberry J. F. The risk of colorectal cancer in ulcerative colitis: a meta-analysis. *Gut*, **48** (2001), 526–35.

12. Dunlop M. G. Guidance on large bowel surveillance for people with two first degree relatives with colorectal cancer or one first degree relative diagnosed with colorectal cancer under 45 years. *Gut*, **51**:suppl. V (2002), 17–20.

13. Aaltonen L. A., Salovaara R., Kristo P., *et al.* Incidence of hereditary non-polyposis colorectal cancer and the feasibility of molecular screening for the disease. *N Engl J Med*, **338** (1998), 1481–7.

14. Ponz de Leon M. Hereditary colon cancer. *Eur J Cancer Prev*, **5** (1996), 372–3.

15. Burt R. W., Bishop D. T., Cannon L. A., *et al.* Dominant inheritance of adenomatous colonic polyps and colorectal cancer. *N Engl J Med*, **312** (1985), 1540–4.

16. Cannon-Albright L. A., Skolnick M. H., Bishop D. T., Lee R. G., and Burt R. W. Common inheritance of susceptibility to colonic adenomatous polyps and associated colorectal cancers. *N Engl J Med*, **319**:9 (1988), 533–7.

17. Lieberman D. A., Weiss D. G., Bond J. H., *et al.* Use of colonoscopy to screen asymptomatic adults for colorectal cancer. Veterans Affairs Cooperative Study Group 380. *N Engl J Med*, **343** (2000), 162–8.

18. Atkin W., Rogers P., Cardwell C., *et al.* Wide variation in adenoma detection rates at screening flexible sigmoidoscopy. *Gastroenterology*, **126**:5 (2004), 1247–56.

19. Neugut A. I., Jacobson J. S., Ahsan H., *et al.* Incidence and recurrence rates of colorectal adenomas: a prospective study. *Gastroenterology*, **108** (1995), 402–8.

20. Winawer S. J., Zauber A. G., Fletcher R. H., *et al.* US Multi-Society Task Force on Colorectal Cancer; American Cancer Society. Guidelines for colonoscopy surveillance after polypectomy: a consensus update by the US Multi-Society Task Force on Colorectal Cancer and the American Cancer Society. *Gastroenterology*, **130** (2006), 1872–85.

21. Vogelstein B., Fearon E. R., Hamilton S. R., *et al.* Genetic alterations during colorectal-tumor development. *N Engl J Med*, **319** (1988), 525–32.

22. ACPGB2I (2001) *Guidelines for the Management of Colorectal Cancer.* Issued by The Association of Coloproctology of Great Britain and Ireland. www.acpgbi.org.uk.

23. McSherry C. K., Cornell G. N., and Glenn F. Carcinoma of the colon and rectum. *Ann Surg*, **169** (1969), 502–9.

24. McDermott F., Hughes E., Pihl E., Milne B., and Price A. Symptom duration and survival prospects in carcinoma of the rectum. *Surg Gynecol Obstet*, **153** (1981), 321–6.

25. McSherry C. K., Grafe W. R. Jr, Perry H. S., and Glenn F. Surgery of the large bowel for emergent conditions: staged vs primary resection. *Arch Surg*, **98** (1969), 749–53.

26. Shallow T. A., Wagner F. B. Jr, and Colcher R. E. Clinical evaluation of 750 patients with colon cancer; diagnostic survey and follow-up covering a fifteen-year period. *Ann Surg*, **142** (1955), 164–75.

27. Ellis B. G., Baig K. M., Senapati A., *et al.* Common modes of presentation of colorectal cancer patients. *Colorect Dis*, **1**:Suppl. 2 (1999), 4.

28. Dodds S., Dodds A., Vakis S., *et al.* The value of various factors associated with rectal bleeding in the diagnosis of colorectal cancer. *Gut*, **44** (1999), A99.

29. Dixon A. R., Thornton-Holmes J., and Cheetham N. M. General practitioner's awareness of colorectal cancer; A 10 year review. *BMJ*, **301** (1990), 152–3.

30. Finan P. J., Ritchie J. K., and Hawley P. R. Synchronous and "early" metachronous carcinomas of the colon and rectum. *Br J Surg*, **74** (1987), 945–7.

31. Barillari P., Ramacciato G., Manetti G., *et al.* Surveillance of colorectal cancer: effectiveness of early detection of intraluminal recurrences on prognosis and survival of patients treated for cure. *Dis Colon Rectum*, **39** (1996), 388–93.

32. DoH. *Manual for Cancer Services*. Gateway ref.3364 (London: Department of Health, 2004).

33. DoH. *Guidance on Commissioning Cancer Services: Improving Outcomes in Colorectal Cancer. The Manual.* (London: Department of Health, 2004).

34. Flood A. and Ewy W. Does practice make perfect? Part II: The relation between volume and outcomes and other hospital characteristics. *Med Care*, **22** (1988), 98–114.

35. Fried B. J., Deber R., and Wilson E. Multidisciplinary teams in health care: lessons from oncology and renal teams. *Healthcare Management FORUM Winter/Hiver*, 1988, 28–34.

36. Haward R., Amir Z., Borrill C., *et al.* Breast cancer teams: the impact of constitution, new cancer workload, and methods of operation on their effectiveness. *BJC*, **89** (2003), 15–22.

37. Wibe A., Eriksen M. T., Syse, A., *et al.* Norwegian rectal cancer group. Effect of hospital caseload on long-term outcome after standardization of rectal cancer surgery at a national level. *Brit J Surg*, **92** (2005), 217–40.

38. Smith J. A., King P. M., Lane R. H., *et al.* Evidence of the effect of 'specialization' on the management, surgical outcome and survival from colorectal cancer in Wessex. *Brit J Surg*, **90** (2003), 583–92.

2

Pathology for the radiologist: pathological insights into colorectal cancer

Philip Quirke

Introduction

For many decades, the management of colorectal cancer was looked upon as the domain of the surgeon. In the last 10 years, this opinion has changed and with the change to multidisciplinary management significant improvements in the management and outcomes of patients have occurred. Initially this has been seen in rectal cancer, but colonic cancer will also benefit by improved radiological and pathological staging. The radiologist and pathologist are central to this process and can learn from each other to gain new insights into their respective fields. First, I will address the rectum and secondly, more briefly, the colon.

The rectum

The success of magnetic resonance imaging in the rectum [1,2] and its increasing resolution has led to an important need for the radiologist to understand the anatomy and gross pathology of rectal cancer. This is best learnt prospectively prior to starting reporting high-resolution MRIs by visiting the pathologist in the cut-up room and then seeing the pathological cross-sectional images at the multidisciplinary team meetings. The radiologist, like the pathologist, will continue to learn and improve with increasing experience of the images. For example, the accuracy of prediction of the circumferential margin is 92% in the hands of an experienced radiologist [3] but only 82% in the large multicentre Mercury study [4]. The accuracy of diagnosis is not reported post chemoradiotherapy but it is likely to be lower. The importance of the circumferential resection margin (CRM) in predicting local recurrence and survival has been shown many times in pathological studies [5,6,7,8,9,10,11,12,13,14,15]. To date, only one series has related the prediction of CRM by MRI to survival [16]. Interestingly, the survival curves are identical to those obtained by pathology. A larger series will be available from the Mercury study and will hopefully reproduce this important finding. Other important radiological features are the T stage of the tumor and the distance of extramural spread as well as the actual distance from the CRM. Both confer prognostic information which is likely to vary from site to site in the rectum as the amount of mesorectum varies between individuals. Radiologists have attempted to predict nodal (N) stage but the literature is disappointing with relatively poor kappa values. Radiologists are also able to predict other features such as extramural vascular invasion and peritoneal involvement. The accuracy of prediction is likely to vary depending on the experience of the radiologist, and the kappa values for such measurements are not currently available. It is possible that with the dynamic nature of MRI a pathological feature may be predicted more frequently or more accurately. This may be the case with extramural venous invasion as flow within the vessel will be interrupted, possibly causing changes to the MRI images. With increasing experience, better techniques and improving strength of MRI machines [17], the accuracy will increase and more knowledge of the gross pathology can only assist this process. This chapter describes the applied anatomy of the mesorectum and anal canal as seen by the pathologist and presents examples of cross-sectional images of rectal cancers to help radiologists interpret their images.

Applied anatomy of the rectum

The anterior and posterior surfaces of an anterior resection total mesorectal excision and an abdominoperineal excision are shown in Figure 2.1. The sphincters have of course been removed on the latter. The key features to appreciate are the large extent of the surgically created CRM and the waist formed when removing the rectum by the standard method. On the anterior surface, the CRM begins at the peritoneal reflection and extends downward to the bottom of the mesorectum and the distal excision margin or, if an abdominoperineal excision, down to the anal skin. Posteriorly, the margin begins much higher near the high tie and extends downward as an enlarging triangle until it reaches the peritoneal reflection where it becomes circumferential. The margin created is very large and must be borne in mind at all times when reporting. Obtaining a clear margin is very important, and a threatened margin is a definite indication for referral for an oncological opinion. The performance of an abdominoperineal excision usually leads to the surgeon following the mesorectal plane and following it onto the sphincters. This leads to a

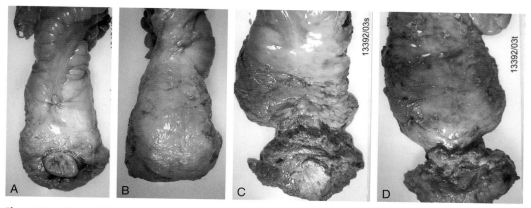

Figure 2.1 **(A) and (B)** show the anterior and posterior surfaces of a total mesorectal excision. In (A), there is early puckering of the peritoneal surface from a mid-rectal cancer. Note the origin of the peritoneum and the small area of the surgical margin anteriorly compared to the large posterior surgical margin. This is an excellent resection removing the entire anatomical structure. **(C) and (D)** show the anterior and posterior surfaces of an abdominoperineal excision. The mesorectum has been removed as well as in (A) and (B) but note the waist caused by the termination of the mesorectum in the low rectum and the surgical plane lies on the sphincter muscles with no removal of the levator ani muscles. This waist is an area for high risk of CRM involvement.

waist which has importance as the radiologist must identify whether the tumor is a pT3 low rectal cancer or through the sphincters. If the surgeon performs the standard AP (abdominoperineal) operation then the margin may be at risk if the tumor is extensively involving the sphincters or is very low in the mesorectum. One further feature of importance is the disposition of the lymph nodes in the rectum. Lymph nodes are usually not found in the ischiorectal fat below the levators. They can, however, be found very low down in the mesorectum, and frequently they abut the posterior mesorectal surface. Involvement may occur either by the surgeon invading the mesorectum and cutting into a metastatic deposit or by invasion of the tumor through the mesorectum and out to the mesorectal fascia leading to an involved margin by extensive tumor spread. An anterior resection showing at least 12 lymph nodes identified with arrows is shown in Figure 2.2. Many of these lymph nodes lie against the circumferential margin and two small lymph nodes are shown right at the base of the mesorectum. Attention should be paid to the iliac and obturator nodes in low rectal cancer as spread may occur outside the usual western planes of surgery. Recent studies suggest that such spread is not a frequent cause of recurrence [18].

It should be borne in mind that the size of the mesorectum varies widely between individuals [19] as does the shape of the pelvic inlet [20]. The former should be

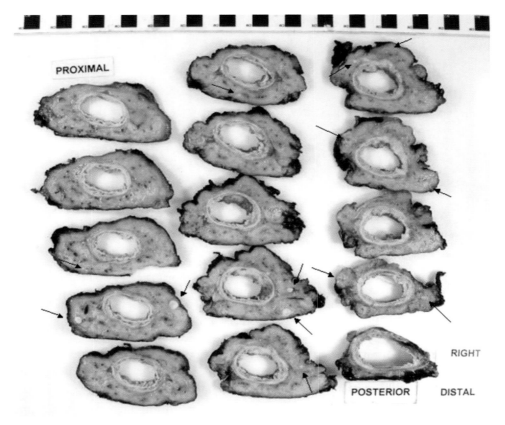

Figure 2.2   Disposition of lymph nodes (arrowed) in a total mesorectal excision many of them lying close to the circumferential margin and extending down into the base of the mesorectum.

borne in mind when reporting rectal cancer. The rectum is oval in shape with less tissue anteriorly and laterally [15] and CRM involvement is expected to be more frequent in this area. The highest rates are seen in the lowest 4 cm of the rectum/anal canal where the mesorectum sharply tapers and the levators fuse to form the external sphincter [15,21].

Pathological features of importance to the radiologist

After identifying the presence of an invasive cancer, the radiologist would usually attempt to T and N stage the tumor. Whilst the T stage is very important, attention has moved to the potential for achieving a clear resection margin by predicting pathological involvement of this margin and measuring the distance to the CRM. The continually improving scanning techniques and increasing experience of radiologists have made MRI a mandatory examination for patients with rectal cancer. Radiologists can also accurately identify the extent of spread from the muscularis propria and can occasionally predict other important pathological features such as extramural vascular invasion and peritoneal involvement. The prediction of large deposits of tumor in lymph nodes is possible by MRI but is far from perfect when taking into account the level of agreement by chance. This is high as around half of all cases are node positive and thus a tossed coin would obtain 50% agreement by chance. Many involved lymph nodes are small and may not be picked up by MRI. Occasionally, very small involved lymph nodes are seen, only a few mm's in size. If the pathologists are using the 6th edition of TNM (TNM6), agreement may be even worse owing to the classification of all round structures as lymph nodes. The 5th edition of TNM uses a definition of tumor nodules greater than 3 mm in size as being lymph nodes. Whilst the evidence for this definition is weak, it does have the advantage of offering a measurable target for the radiologist and this may increase pathologist/radiologist agreement. The UK, Belgium and much of Scandinavia have refused to move to TNM6 as the evidence base is inadequate for the new classification of lymph node and venous invasion, and the interobserver variability is poor [22].

Surgical circumferential resection margin

The circumferential resection margin (CRM) is an extensive surgically created plane of dissection produced during the removal of the rectum from its surroundings. The largest area of CRM is posterior, and a full 360° circumferential margin appears below the peritoneal reflection. The frequency of histological involvement of the CRM is strongly associated with local recurrence and poor survival. Tumor within 1 mm of the surgically created margin greatly increases the risk of recurrence. One study showed that the risk is lesser, but still high, at 2 mm [11]; but other investigations have not confirmed this finding [5,7,9,10,12]. With standard surgery, 36% of all patients and 25% of those undergoing a curative operation showed CRM involvement [5,7,9]. In our centre, the frequency of involvement of the CRM varied substantially between individual surgeons [9].

In studies where mesorectal excision has been taught and adopted, the CRM involvement rate has also fallen. In a Norwegian study involving 686 patients, this rate fell to 9.4% [14], and in the Dutch study where 656 patients were treated by TME alone the frequency was 18.3% [23]. Two other UK Medical Research

Council Trials CLASICC and CR07 have reported frequencies of CRM involvement of 14% [24] and 11% [25].

Distance to the CRM

Several studies, including our own series, have shown that the distance to the CRM is related to outcome. This is also a continuous variable, the risk of death increasing with every mm closer to the CRM. This measurement will also be affected by the quality of surgery. Thus, the absolute distance of tumor from the CRM should also be quoted by the radiologist.

Distance from the muscularis propria

The distance tumor spreads from the muscularis propria is an important prognostic feature. For every mm of spread from the muscularis propria there is a worsening of 5-year survival. However the mesorectum is not a symmetrical structure. There is less mesorectum situated anteriorly and anterolaterally than posteriorly, thus, it is likely that prognosis will be affected by the quadrant of the tumor as well as the depth. Nine millimeters of spread in the former will lead to a higher risk of incomplete excision than 9 mm in the posterior mesorectum. The size of the mesorectum also varies meaning that in one individual spread of tumor, 15 mm from the muscularis propria, may lead to an involved margin whereas in another with a tumor situated posteriorly in the rectum the tumor may be less than halfway through the mesorectal fat. The real importance of these features also depends on the surgeon and how effectively the rectum is removed.

Peritoneal and extramural vascular invasion

It is a fact that a good radiologist can sometimes identify peritoneal involvement and extramural vascular invasion. A radiologist should always look for the signs of these features of poor prognosis. They may occasionally tip the balance toward more aggressive therapy by the multidisciplinary team. Peritoneal involvement can be seen presenting with a gull's-wing appearance, a broad invasive front, or both; examples are shown in Figure 2.3. Occasionally, a double gull's wing may be seen and an example is shown in Figure 2.4. Pathologically, vascular invasion can be seen in the muscularis propria as thin finger-like projections through the muscle

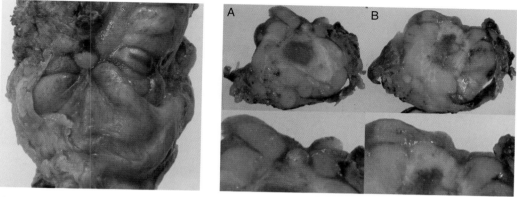

Figure 2.3   Peritoneal involvement showing the typical gull's wing sign in A with a magnified picture of the area and arising below it in B, an area of broad-based peritoneal involvement with a magnified picture.

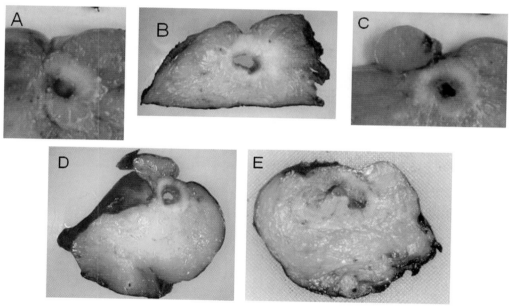

Figure 2.4   More examples of peritoneal involvement with different degrees of the gull's wing sign A, B, and C with D showing a double gull's wing. E shows broad-based peritoneal involvement.

in the areas where vessels are known to penetrate. Several foci may be present increasing the certainty of the diagnosis; examples are shown in Figure 2.5. The accuracy of the prediction of these factors has not been reported but this data should be available from the Mercury project.

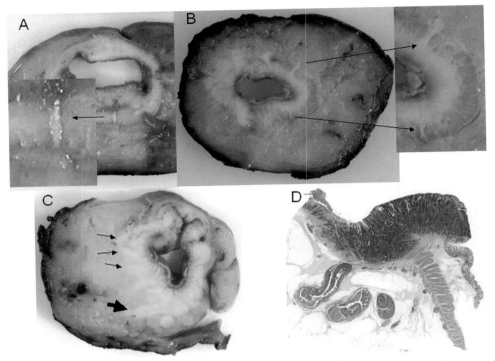

Figure 2.5 **(A) very early stage of venous involvement with tumor within a vein penetrating the muscularis propria. (B) early intramural venous invasion extending through the muscularis propria but also associated with more bulky extramural vascular invasion. (C) varying degrees of extramural vascular invasion with large vein invasion at the bottom. An involved lymph node is also apparent. (D) histological section showing only large vein extramural vascular invasion.**

A feature that has not been reported radiologically is the presence of a pushing or infiltrating border. The correlation between pathology and radiology is unknown but there is potential for prognostic information in this feature. Radiology can also identify mucinous tumors but again the prognostic value of this feature has not been reported for the preoperative situation.

Low rectal cancer

Recently, we have reported major problems with the operations performed for low rectal cancer. We have shown that in operations with removal of the sphincters, a high rate of tumor involvement of the circumferential margin (up to one-third of patients) and frequent perforation (16%) was seen in Leeds [15]

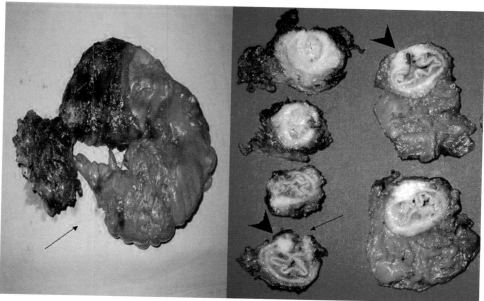

Figure 2.6 Abdominoperineal excision showing an anterior perforation below the mesorectum in the area of the sphincters. The mesorectal excision is very good but the surgical plane has led to perforation in the area of the tumor (arrow), and on the cross-sections the perforation can also be seen directly adjacent to the tumor. The tumor is involving the circumferential margin (arrow heads).

and in a major Dutch trial [23]. The rate of CRM involvement is frequently more than double in APEs than ARs and the rate of perforation 4–6 times more frequent. This is because of the difficulty of operating in the low pelvis via an abdominal incision and the anatomy of the low rectum. An example of a sphincteric perforation and adjacent circumferential margin involvement is shown in Figure 2.6.

The mesorectum ends abruptly just above the levators. The surgeon follows the mesorectal plane and moves onto the insertion of the levators. The surgeon incises the levators where it fuses with the external sphincter leading to the "apple core appearance" of the standard surgical AP specimen. Thus, the radiologist needs to be aware of the surgical planes that the surgeon follows to advise them of the potential for a complete excision. There is variation in the technique of removal of the sphincters; in Stockholm, T. Holm from the Karolinska Hospital removed a cylindrical specimen using a different technique. The abdominal dissection is performed first down to the level of the prostate or the posterior fornix of the vagina. Then the patient is flipped over and the anal and low rectal dissection is completed from below. In this operation, there is a much greater degree of dissection from below, and the planes are readily visualized allowing more control over the plane of excision. The levators can be removed from below at their origin near to the pelvic wall allowing them to be kept applied to the surgical specimen and thus forming a wider plane of excision that should reduce the frequency of CRM involvement. This approach should also reduce or even abolish tumor perforation as the surgeon has greater access and can identify planes more easily. This operation will not increase the tissue removable anteriorly but will give greater clearance laterally and posteriorly. The potential for greater side effects is present and the benefits of this wider operation must be assessed in practice.

Education

It is important that radiologists become familiar with the pathology of their cases and new educational initiatives are required. With Professor Sir Mike Brady of Oxford University and Dr. Gina Brown of the Royal Marsden, we have been funded by the NCRI bioinformatics initiative to create an integrated radiology/pathology platform and the first cases can be seen at www.virtualpathology.leeds.ac.uk/teaching. Professor Sir Mike Brady is also working with this material to develop new approaches to the assessment of the MRI and pathology images. To date, he has developed a program for the automatic removal of the luminal and mesorectal planes and their 3D display as well as the 3D reconstruction of the specimens as shown in the figures. We will also develop programs for the assessment of response to chemotherapy and its comparison to pathology and automatic structure identification comparing MRI images with the resultant pathology.

Postchemoradiotherapy changes

The pathological changes after short-course radiation have been well described by Nagtegaal and the Dutch group [26]. There is a minor degree of downstaging in some individuals and the lymphocytic reaction is reduced. The accuracy of predicting involvement of the CRM should not be affected but there is no prospective data to prove this. Much greater changes are seen following long-course radiotherapy and radiochemotherapy where substantial regression up to complete response may be seen. Difficulties arise for the radiologists because of the fibrosis, necrosis, and mucin lakes that are formed post treatment. It is not possible for a radiologist to state there has been a definite complete response because single tumor cells may remain. The size of the change between two scans can be reported and an indication of the bulk of the residual tumor-bearing area can be given. Quantitative measurement of the reduction in bulk and the relationship to unresectable structures, the mesorectal fascia, and levators should be given. The histological appearance of tumors post chemoradiotherapy are shown in Figure 2.7 and the correlation of the macroscopic pathology to the haematoxylin and eosin sections in Figure 2.8. Post chemoradiotherapy, the CRM maintains

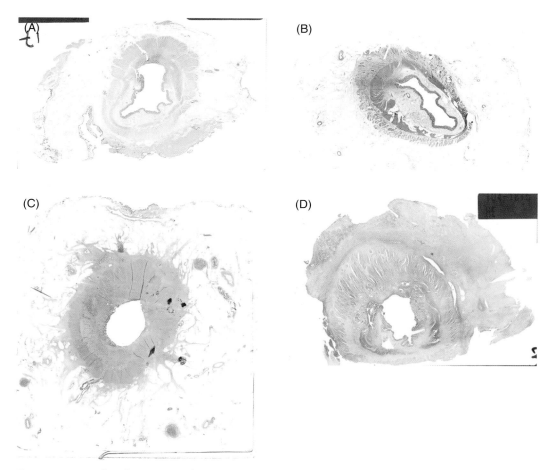

Figure 2.7   Examples of response to chemoradiotherapy. (A) complete response with no residual tumor; only a small area of residual mucosal ulceration. (B) and (C) good responses with only a few tumor cells visible on microscopy. (D) moderate response the tumor bulk has been reduced, and there is a fibrotic reaction but substantial numbers of tumor cells are still present. Arrows show site of tumor of residual ulceration.

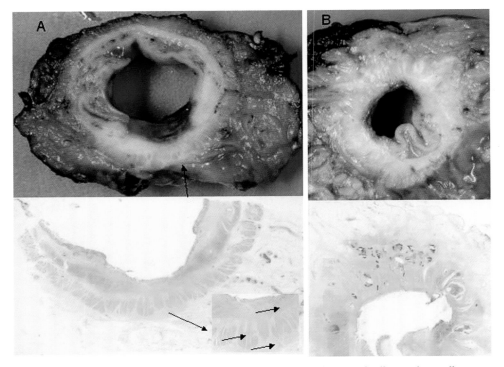

Figure 2.8   (A) good response. Macroscopically, there are two small areas of yellow and a small amount of fibrosis but there are microscopic areas of tumor present. (B) moderate response. Whilst there has been extensive destruction of tumor, there are still easily findable tumor deposits as well as the areas of pink/blue necrosis that show up as yellow areas on the macroscopic specimen.

its importance for the prediction of outcome with several studies reporting its impact on survival [27,28,29,30]. The effect appears to be the same as without chemoradiotherapy. Complete surgical excision is a key feature of success in advanced cases. Regression grading does impact on survival with a complete response having a better outcome than microscopic disease and the latter doing better than moderate, mild, or no regression [31,32,33,34].

The multidisciplinary team meetings

The radiologist and pathologist are key members of the multidisciplinary team (MDT) meetings. Radiologists should expect digital pictures of the surgical specimens to be projected. These should include the anterior and posterior surfaces and the cross-sectional images. These images will allow high-quality correlation between the radiological predictions and the histopathology, and can act as a useful learning process for both disciplines.

The colon

The anatomy of the colon is more complex and variable than the rectum and individual variation is poorly documented. The general relationships to other organs and structures are well defined, but important surgically created planes are less well described and probably not appreciated by radiologist and pathologist alike.

What key features should we consider? The peritoneal covering of the colon is critical in that both the colon and its mesentery are covered in this boundary and penetration of it allows spread outside the surgical field. Surgically, the creation of a retroperitoneal margin in the cecum/ascending colon is important and the descending colon may have a retroperitoneal margin, albeit of variable size, as shown in Figure 2.9. The existence of the mesocolon is hardly appreciated and the importance of removing this intact is not realized. Examples of an intact removal and a poor removal of the mesocolon of the right and left colons are shown in Figures 2.10 and 2.11, respectively. The sigmoid colon has a mesentery of variable length and its origin is variable leading to difficulties of definition from the rectum.

The importance of the peritoneal surface has been highlighted in the significant work by Neil Shepherd [35,36] but it is still too little appreciated. The true frequency of peritoneal invasion in the colon is not well established but is certainly over 30% and may be much higher. Since it is possible to detect advanced peritoneal involvement in the rectum by the gull's wing or double gull's wing sign described by Brown, can we see it in the colon? Yes, it is a prominent pathological feature just like in the rectum; but, can it be accurately predicted by the radiologist? If so, would neoadjuvant or intraperitoneal therapy offer any benefit? The importance of the quality of colonic surgery has not been appreciated. The mesentery of the colon – whilst smaller, varying by anatomical site, and much more irregular than the rectum – is an important structure that drains the tumor and contains important structures such as lymphatics, lymph nodes, veins, and nerves. All these structures which can be pathways to metastatic spread. All too often this structure is either damaged or the length of excision compromised by inadequate surgery. Local recurrence of right-sided colon cancer is more frequent than that of left-sided colon cancer. This may be in part caused by the existence of

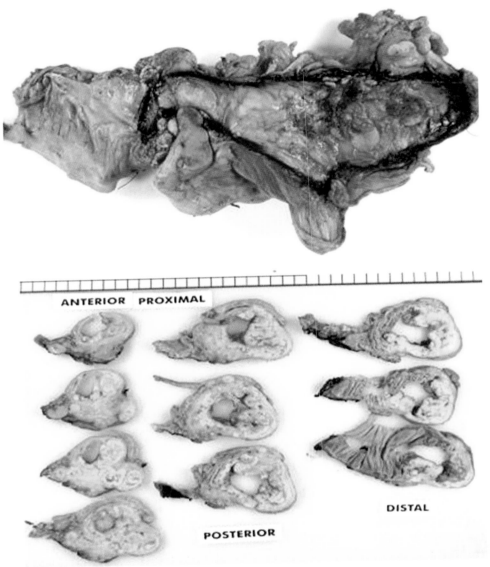

Figure 2.9   Surgically created retroperitoneal margin on the right side of the colon. This is outlined by India ink. The cross-sections of the ascending colon show tumor extending to the deep surgical margin.

the diamond-shaped surgical margin created by removal of the cecum/ascending colon from the psoas muscle and other retroperitoneal surfaces. The size of this area varies between individuals. The presence of a large retroperitoneal surface opens up the possibility of surgical margin involvement which has been reported at 10% [37].

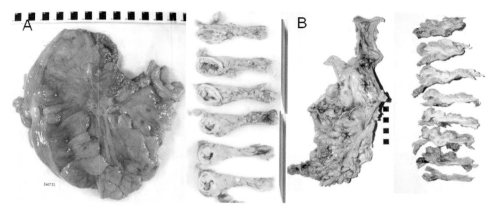

Figure 2.10   Two examples of right hemicolectomies. In A, the mesocolon has been removed almost in its entiety. In B, only a small proportion of the mesocolon has been removed.

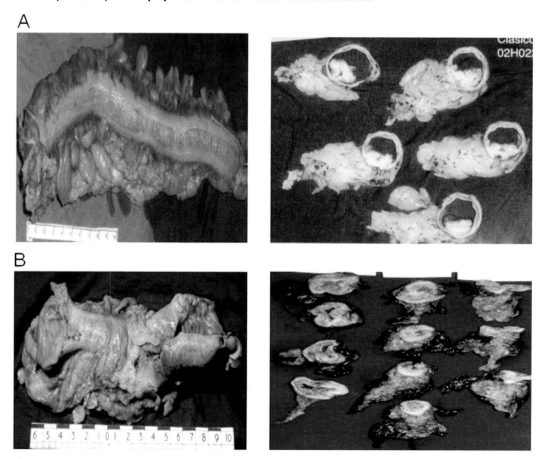

Figure 2.11   Two examples of left-sided colonic surgery. In A, the mesocolon has been removed intact whereas in B the mesocolon has been badly damaged.

What lessons for the radiologist in the colon?

Many of the features that are visible in the rectum should also be reportable in the colon. The anatomy is complicated; and obtaining the right axis in a convoluted structure is more challenging; but with new software it should be possible to recreate the colon in any plane. What features should you be looking for? Involvement of the likely retroperitoneal margin in the ascending colon may be visible. Since prediction of involvement in the mesorectum is accurate, this too may prove to be so. The measurement of extramural spread has also been identified as accurate in the Mercury study and this is related to prognosis in colon as well as rectum. The presence of gull's wings may indicate an advanced tumor with peritoneal involvement, and perforation may be readily apparent from gas under the diaphragm. In future, nodal spread and extramural vascular invasion may also be reportable. The key is to look hard and take a positive and not nihilistic approach to a disease that is twice as common as rectal cancer. New trials of neoadjuvant chemotherapy are needed for colon cancer but these must be based on effective staging. Radiologists are potentially on the edge of helping to select such patients and will play a major role in driving forward new modalities of treatment in colon cancer. They should work with pathologists to solve this important clinical problem. Accurate preoperative staging of colonic tumors would bring about much better management of these patients.

Acknowledgments

Professor Quirke is supported by Yorkshire Cancer Research. www.virtualpathology.leeds.ac.uk is supported by grants from the Department of Health and NCRI. The ideas on colon cancer have been derived from the MRC-supported Classic trial and from discussions in Stockholm with T. Holm and P. O. Nystrom. My knowledge of radiology is indebted to Dr. Gina Brown.

REFERENCES

1. Blomqvist, L., Rubio, C., Holm, T., Machado, M., and Hindmarsh, T. Rectal adenocarcinoma: assessment of tumour involvement of the lateral resection margin by MRI of the resected specimen. *Br J Radiol*, **72** (1999), 18–23.
2. Brown, G., Richards, C. J., Newcombe, R. G., *et al*. Rectal carcinoma: thin-section MR imaging for staging in 28 patients. *Radiology*, **211** (1999), 215–22.

3. Brown, G., Radcliffe, A. G., Newcombe, R. G., *et al*. Preoperative assessment of prognostic factors in rectal cancer using high resolution magnetic resonance imaging. *Br J Surg*, **90** (2003), 355–64.

4. Extramural depth of tumour invasion at their section MR in patients with rectal cancer: Results of the mercury trial. *Radiology*, **243** (2007), 132–9.

5. Quirke, P., Durdey, P., Dixon, M. F., and Williams, N. S. Local recurrence of rectal adenocarcinoma is caused by inadequate surgical resection: histopathological study of lateral tumour spread and surgical excision. *Lancet*, **ii** (1986), 996–9.

6. Ng, I. O., Luk, I. S., Yuen, S. T., *et al*. Surgical lateral clearance in resected rectal carcinomas: a multivariate analysis of clinicopathological features. *Cancer*, **71** (1993), 1972–6.

7. Adam, I. J., Mohamdee, M. O., Martin, I. G., *et al*. Role of circumferential margin involvement in the local recurrence of rectal cancer. *Lancet*, **344** (1994), 707–11.

8. de Haas-Koch, D. F., Baeten, C. G. M. I., Jager, J. J., *et al*. Prognostic significance of radial margins of clearance in rectal carcinoma. *Br J Surg*, **83** (1996), 781–5.

9. Birbeck, K. F., Macklin, C. P., Tiffin, N. J., *et al*. Rates of circumferential margin involvement vary between surgeons and predict outcomes in rectal cancer surgery. *Ann Surg*, **235**:4 (2002), 449–57.

10. Wibe, A., Rendedal, P. R., Svensson, E., Norstein, J., Eide, T. J., Myrvold, H. E., Soreide, O. on behalf of the Norwegian Rectal Cancer Group. Prognostic significance of the circumferential resection margin following total mesorectal excision for rectal cancer. *Br J Surg*, **89** (2002), 327–34.

11. Nagtegaal, I. D., Marijnen, C. A. M., Kranenbarg, E. K., van de Velde, C. J. H., and van Krieken, J. H. J. M. Circumferential margin involvement is still an important predictor of local recurrence in rectal carcinoma. Not one millimetre but two millimetres is the limit. *Am J Surg Pathol*, **26** (2002), 350–7.

12. Maughan, N. J., Morris, E., Craig, S. C., *et al*. Analysis of Northern and Yorkshire Cancer Registry Data 1995–2001. *J Pathol*, **201**:suppl. (2003), 18A.

13. Martling, A., Singnomklao, T., Holm, T., Rutqvist, L. E., and Cedermark, B. Prognostic significance of both surgical and pathological assessment of curative resection for rectal cancer. *Br J Surg*, **91** (2004), 1040–5.

14. Wibe, A., Syse, A., Andersen, E., Tredi, S., Myrvold, H. E., Soreide, O. on behalf of the Norwegian Rectal Cancer Group. Oncological outcomes after total mesorectal excision for cure for cancer of the lower rectum: anterior resection vs abdominoperineal resection. *Dis Colon Rectum* **47** (2004), 48–58.

15. Marr, R., Birbeck, K., Garvican, J., *et al*. The modern abdominoperineal excision: the next challenge after total mesorectal excision. *Ann Surg*, **242**:1 (July 2005), 74–82.

16. Martling, A., Holm, T., Bremmner, S., *et al*. Prognostic value of preoperative magnetic resonance imaging of the pelvis in rectal cancer. *Br J Surg*, **90** (2003), 1422–8.

17. Kim, C. K., Kim, S. H., Chun, K. H., *et al*. Preoperative staging of rectal cancer: accuracy of 3-Tesla magnetic resonance imaging. *Eur Radiol*, **16** (2006), 972–80.

18. Syk, E., Torkzad, M. R., Blomqvist, L., Ljungqvist, O., and Glimelius, B. Radiological findings do not support lateral residual tumour as a major cause of local recurrence of rectal cancer. *Br J Surg*, **93** (2006), 113–19.

19. Torkzad, M. R. and Blomqvist, L. The mesorectum: morphometric assessment with magnetic resonance imaging. *Eur Radiol*, **15** (2005), 1184–91.

20. Boyle, K. M., Petty, D., Chalmers, A. G., *et al.* MRI assessment of the bony pelvis may help predict resectability of the rectal cancer. *Colorect Dis*, **7** (2005), 232–40.

21. Nagtegaal, I. D., van de Velde, C. J. H., Marijnen, C. A. M., van Krieken, J. H. J. M., and Quirke, P. for the pathology review committee and the cooperative clinical investigators of the Dutch Colorectal Cancer Group. Low rectal cancer; a call for a change of approach in abdominoperineal resection. *J Clin Oncol*, **23**:36 (2005), 9257–64.

22. Howarth, S. M., Morgan, J. M., and Williams, G. T. The new (6th edition) TNM classification of colorectal cancer a stage too far. *Gut*, **53** (2004), A21.

23. Kapiteijn, E., Marijnen, C. A. M., Nagtegaal, I. D., Putten, H., Steup, W. H., Wiggers, T., Rutten, H., Pahlman, L., Glimelius, B., van Krieken, H. J. M., Leer, J. W. H., van de Velde, C. J. H. for the Dutch Colorectal Cancer Group. Preoperative radiotherapy combined with total mesorectal excision for respectable rectal cancer. *N Engl J Med*, **345** (2001), 638–46.

24. Guillou, P., Quirke, P., Thorpe, H., Walker, J., Jayne, D., Smith, A. M. H., Heath, R. M., Brown, J. M. for the MRC CLASICC Trial Group. Short-term endpoints of conventional versus laparoscopic assisted surgery in patients with colorectal cancer (MRC CLASICC trial): multicentre, randomised controlled trial. *Lancet*, **365** (2005), 1718–26.

25. Quirke, P., Sebag-Montefiore, D., Steele, R., Khanna, S., Monson, J., Holliday, A., Thompson, L., Griffiths, G., Stephanie, R., on behalf of all the CR07 participants. Local recurrence after rectal cancer resection is strongly related to the plane of surgical dissection and is further reduced by pre-operative short course radiotherapy. *J Clin Oncol*, **24** (2006), Part I suppl 1495.

26. Nagtegaal, I. D., Marijnen, C. A. M., Kranebarg, E. K., *et al.* Pathology Review Committee. Short term preoperative radiotherapy interferes with the determination of pathological parameters in rectal cancer. *J Pathol*, **197** (2002), 20–7.

27. Mawdsley, S., Glynne-Jones, R., Grainger, J., *et al.* Can the histopathological assessment of the circumferential margin following pre-operative pelvic chemo-radiotherapy for T3/4 rectal cancer predict for three year disease free survival? *Int J Radiation Oncol*, **63** (2005), 745–52.

28. Sebag-Montefiore, D., Glynne-Jones, R., Mortensen, N., *et al.* Pooled analysis of outcome measures including the histopathological R0 resection rate after preoperative chemoradiation for locally advanced rectal cancer. *Colorect Dis*, **7**:suppl. 22 (2005), A20.

29. Sebag-Montefiore, D., Hingorani, M., Cooper, R., and Chesser, P. Circumferential resection margin status predicts outcome after pre-operative chemoradiation for locally advanced rectal cancer. http://www.asco.org/ac/1,003,12-002636-0018-0036-00190010208.00.asp.

30. Luna-Perez, P., Bustos-Cholico, E., Alvarado, I., *et al*. Prognostic significance of circumferential margin involvement in rectal adenocarcinoma treated with preoperative chemoradiotherapy and low anterior resection. *J Surg Oncol*, **90** (2005), 20–5.

31. Rodel, C., Martus, P., Papadoupolos, T., *et al*. Prognostic significance of tumour regression after preoperative chemoradiotherapy for rectal cancer. *J Clin Oncol*, **23** (2005), 8688–96.

32. Mandard, A. M., Dalibard, F., Mandard, J. C., *et al*. Pathological assessment of tumour regression after preoperative chemoradiotherapy of esophageal carcinoma. Clinicopathological correlations. *Cancer*, **73** (1994), 2680–6.

33. Dworak, O., Keilholtz, L., and Hoffmann, A. Pathological features of rectal cancer after preoperative radiochemotherapy. *Int J Colorect Dis*, **12** (1997), 19–23.

34. Bouzourene, H., Bosman, F. T., Seelentag, W., Matter, M., and Coucke, P. Importance of tumour regression assessment in predicting outcome in patients with locally advanced rectal carcinoma who are treated with preoperative radiotherapy. *Cancer*, **94** (2002), 1121–30.

35. Petersen, V. C., Baxter, K. J., Love, S. B., and Shepherd, N. A. Identification of objective pathological prognostic determinants and models of prognosis in Dukes' B colon cancer. *Gut*, **51** (2002), 65–9.

36. Ludeman, L. and Shepherd, N. A. Serosal involvement in gastrointestinal cancer: its assessment and significance. *Histopathology*, **47** (2005), 123–31.

37. Bateman, A. C., Carr, N. J., and Warren, B. F. The retroperitoneal surface in distal caecal and proximal ascending colon carcinoma: the Cinderella surgical margin? *J Clin Pathol*, **58**:4 (April 2005), 426–8.

3

Screening for colorectal cancer

Steve Halligan

Introduction

It is well worthwhile screening for colorectal cancer. Several factors underpin this statement. The disease is common – approximately 5% of the Western world will develop colorectal cancer – and also fatal in approximately 50% of those who have the disease. This is because symptoms frequently do not appear until the disease is relatively advanced (and therefore incurable), and also because symptoms are ignored by patients. This is because the symptoms of colorectal cancer are non-specific and, as a result, common in the general population. For example, the vast majority of people suffering a change in bowel habit and rectal bleeding do not have cancer. Even if they do, such symptoms are frequently ignored.

It is not enough for a disease to be common and fatal for it to be considered a good candidate for screening; it is important that effective curative treatment is available for those in whom a diagnosis of established cancer is made by screening at an early stage. With this in mind, survival rate for patients with a Dukes' A colorectal cancer is at least 85% versus 40% or worse for those with a Dukes' C tumor.

In the majority of cases, colorectal cancer arises from pre-existing benign adenomatous polyps (via the "adenoma–carcinoma" sequence), and, even then, malignant transformation is believed to take an average of 10 to 15 years. Because of this, there are two related but different approaches to screening programs for colorectal cancer. First, it is possible to target early cancers, so that these patients can benefit from the enhanced survival associated with timely treatment. However, this type of approach, while it may reduce mortality from colorectal cancer (as we shall see later), does nothing to impact on the incidence of the disease. Treatment costs are high – patients with cancer will need to have a colonic resection – and testing will have to be relatively frequent to pick up cancers (especially if the test is relatively insensitive). Furthermore, positive patients may be unduly anxious because they are aware that cancer is the target.

An alternative approach is to target the precursor adenoma because there is indirect evidence that removing these polyps prevents the development of subsequent cancer by interrupting the adenoma–carcinoma sequence. Thus, patients ordinarily destined to develop cancer are prevented from ever doing so by the screening program and the incidence of the disease is reduced (as opposed to schemes that aim to detect cancer only). Also, the costs of treating (and palliating) cancer are largely eliminated, as is surgery-related morbidity and mortality. Because malignant transformation takes many years in most cases, screening can be less frequent than schemes that aim to detect established cancer. Also, screenees who test positive may be less anxious because they are aware that the target lesions (i.e., polyps) are not cancerous. However, polyps are more difficult to detect than cancers, because they are small, and a vast number of polyps need to be removed to prevent a single cancer; this adds to expense.

Thus, there are two different approaches: early detection of established cancer or prevention of cancer by prophylactic polypectomy. All screening programs essentially combine these two approaches, but to varying degrees.

There are also factors that confound easy screening. Unlike cervical, breast, or prostatic programs, both sexes need to be screened, roughly doubling the cost of the program. Like colorectal cancer, lung cancer affects men and women but it is well recognized that smoking is a major risk factor that outweighs all others. As a result, only smokers need to be screened. In contrast, at least 75% of patients who develop colorectal cancer have no specific risk factors that are identifiable in advance. Unfortunately, this means that mass population screening is necessary in order to impact significantly on the disease. Indeed, the most significant risk factor for most people is merely age – the older you are, the more likely you are to develop colorectal cancer. Clearly, having to target everyone above a certain age adds to the expense of any screening program. In addition, the vast majority of adenomas are destined never to become malignant, but there is essentially no efficient way to distinguish in advance those that will from those that will not. This essentially means that all adenomas detected can be regarded as potential cancers and should be removed. However, 30% of the population aged 60 years and older have an adenoma, with the result that many screenees will need polypectomy. Again, this adds to the expense of the program, not least because endoscopy is a skilled procedure currently in short supply. Furthermore, endoscopic polypectomy is unfortunately associated with a small but significant morbidity and even mortality. A fairly blunt instrument with which to identify those adenomas that are most likely to become malignant is measurement of their maximal transverse diameter; the larger the adenoma, the more likely it is to become malignant given time. Indeed, the larger the adenoma, the greater the risk of established cancer within it; 1% at 1 cm or less versus 50% at 2 cm or more.

Which test to use?

Perhaps, one of the major problems with screening for colorectal cancer and adenomas is that there are potentially a plethora of tests to choose from. Each has its own strengths and weaknesses, and some pundits believe that continual and prolonged discussion, turf-battles, and disagreement around which test to employ has delayed the introduction of national programs and has ultimately cost lives.

As intimated already, it is important to understand what the program is trying to achieve and to distinguish those tests that aim predominantly to detect early cancers that are amenable to treatment, from those that target the adenoma, the aim of which is to prevent cancer ever developing. As stated above, most patients with cancer have no identifiable risk factors in advance of their disease and age is the best independent risk factor. The risk of cancer increases exponentially with age: 50% of new diagnoses of colorectal cancer are made after the age of 75 years. Therefore, most screening programs are targeted at older individuals. Where the aim is to prevent cancer by polypectomy, it makes sense to target a somewhat younger age group because adenoma development (especially in the left colon) tends to plateau after the age of 60 years. It is therefore sensible to administer a test that predominantly detects adenomas at a time when most adenomas have developed (in those patients destined to do so) but before invasive cancer has become established. Also, older screenees are most at risk from adverse events associated with colonoscopy, about which more later.

Fecal occult blood testing

Cancers tend to bleed and it is this phenomenon on which the success of fecal occult blood testing (FOBT) is based – FOBT detects blood in feces. Problems with FOBT are well rehearsed – cancers frequently only bleed intermittently and so multiple testing is needed to enhance sensitivity (conventionally three samples). Even when multiple stool samples are obtained, overall sensitivity is approximately

40% for cancer; i.e., 60% of cancer established at the time of testing is missed. Other factors can cause false-positive tests, e.g., ingestion of red meat, and so when positive, the test may have to be repeated with dietary restriction. Overall, patients with a repeatedly positive FOBT test have a 10% chance of having cancer and a 30%–40% chance of having a large polyp (usually an adenoma 2 cm or larger since these bleed more than smaller polyps). It follows that about 50%–60% of patients with a positive FOBT will be normal, so that FOBT has relatively low specificity for cancer in those that have tested positive. A major disadvantage of FOBT is that it is an *indirect* test – the tumor or polyp itself is not directly imaged. Rather, FOBT targets an epiphenomenon and another test is needed to confirm the diagnosis of neoplasia (and to remove it if bleeding is caused by a polyp). At the time of writing, the UK government is implementing a national screening program based on FOBT testing, with colonoscopy the preferred follow-up diagnostic test in the 2% of patients who will test positive. Also, bleeding is a characteristic of cancers and very large adenomas. The vast majority of adenomas do not bleed and, as a consequence, FOBT is poorly suited to a screening program that aims to prevent cancer.

However, despite all of the problems described above, FOBT is the only screening test for which there is randomized controlled evidence that demonstrates reduced disease-specific mortality from colorectal cancer when the test is applied to the relevant population. Many large-scale trials of several thousand patients have all shown a reduction in disease-specific mortality [1,2,3]. Meta-analysis of these trials, performed on data from 329 642 screenees, found the reduction in colorectal cancer mortality to be 16% overall for those who were invited to be screened, with a figure of 23% for those who actually attended for screening [4]. The importance of these data cannot be stressed strongly enough. They represent level 1a evidence that screening for colorectal cancer saves lives. Such hard, randomized data does not exist for lung or prostate cancer for example. Randomization is crucial in studies of the effect of screening interventions because this methodology avoids biases, such as lead-time and length-time bias, which artificially enhance the apparent benefits of screening in case-control studies. A description of such biases is beyond the remit of this article but excellent reviews are available [5].

When randomized evidence of efficacy is coupled with the fact that FOBT is relatively cheap to administer (because the test is generally posted to the patient, performed at home, then posted back and read at a central laboratory), it is not difficult to understand why health policymakers are in favor of it. It should also be borne in mind that FOBT can be combined in a program with some of the other tests described below. For example, the relatively low sensitivity of FOBT can be tackled to some extent by more frequent administration. The UK government has implemented and completed two pilot FOBT screening sites of approximately 1 m screenees each. The aim was not to determine if FOBT screening works (we know that it does), but rather to examine whether it is feasible to deliver in practice. The results suggest that it is and the intention is to begin a national screening program in 2006 for individuals aged 60 to 69 years, rolling out to cover the entire UK by 2009. The estimated cost is £37.5 million for the first 2 years.

At this point, it is useful to consider what might happen to "fellow-travellers" in an FOBT program (or indeed any other program). Screening programs aim to save lives by detecting (or preventing) cancer. But, e.g., for every individual screened with cancer detected by an FOBT program, there are 499 "fellow-travellers," who derive no benefit, and who may actually be harmed. Raffle has elegantly disentangled this [6], and it is worthwhile considering the implications: for every 100 000 individuals screened with FOBT, 3269 will test positive and will need retesting, with all of the anxiety that this entails. Ultimately, 1936 will be persistently positive and will need colonoscopy (or barium enema/CT colonography) to determine the reason why. Of these, 35 will have cancer detected and their life will be prolonged; these patients are the "holy-grail" of the screening program. However, 82 will have cancer detected from which they will die because it is incurable. For these 82 patients, the screening program has only meant that they are aware of their illness (and miserable) for longer than if they had never been screened. Of 1625 negative colonoscopies, 6 will have cancer that was missed (because no test is perfect, even colonoscopy), and they will die also. A further 8 patients without cancer will suffer serious complications from the procedure (e.g., perforation, bleeding, death). Furthermore, an estimated 180 to 540 will have polyps and so on detected that need treating, and about 30 will enter long-term follow-up regimes, with all of the associated expense and inconvenience. Of the 98 064 patients whose FOBT was negative, 55 will develop symptomatic cancer within 2 years, because FOBT is relatively insensitive for established cancer [6].

It can be seen, therefore, that there is a lot of "noise" around the 35 patients who benefit from the program in this example. The aim of this is not to be pessimistic about screening for colorectal cancer – the case for screening is incontrovertible – it is merely to point out facts of which we, as doctors, need to be aware.

Endoscopy

Both colonoscopy and flexible sigmoidoscopy have been promoted as viable approaches to screening for colorectal cancer. In contrast to FOBT, endoscopy is very sensitive for even the smallest adenomas and has a sensitivity for cancer that likely exceeds 95%. This is because bowel lesions are visualized directly by the endoscopist, as opposed to the indirect approach of FOBT. As a consequence, endoscopy is well suited to schemes that aim to detect adenomas and so prevent cancer by polypectomy. However, colonoscopy in particular is expensive, resource intensive, and difficult to master – a recent UK audit suggested that cecal intubation rates were of the order of 50% overall [7]. Colonoscopy-associated adverse events are also well recognized, and are especially related to the sedation usually necessary for the procedure to be comfortable and acceptable. Moreover, these adverse events occur most frequently in older patients, who are most at risk from colorectal cancer. The small mortality associated with colonoscopy could potentially become significant in the context of a screening program where colonoscopy was used as the primary screening test. For example, it has been estimated that 12 patients could die each year in a UK national screening program that used colonoscopy to further investigate screenees whose FOBT is persistently positive [8].

Because of this, it has been suggested that flexible sigmoidoscopy is a more realistic alternative overall. It is safer than colonoscopy because heavy sedation is not required and the left colon is less at risk of perforation during the procedure than the right. It is also much less technically demanding than total colonoscopy and can be performed easily by non-medical staff, given appropriate training. Most cancers and adenomas are left-sided and therefore within reach of the instrument. Modeling has shown that a single flexible sigmoidoscopy at age 55 years would identify those patients who have developed adenomas, enable these to be removed, and so prevent subsequent left-sided cancer [9]. Flexible sigmoidoscopy would also identify early cancers in asymptomatic patients, most of which are left-sided, and also determine indirectly those who may be most at risk of right-sided cancer beyond the reach of the instrument by using left-sided adenomas as a surrogate marker, all within a relatively safe and cost-effective paradigm [8]. Detractors complain that using flexible sigmoidoscopy in a screening program is akin to performing mammography on a single breast because the whole colon is not imaged. However, these arguments ignore the special conditions that apply to screening programs; "patients" are asymptomatic (i.e., the vast majority are not ill) and it is important that they come to as little harm as possible as a consequence of the test used. A more valid criticism is that a tendency to increased right-sided cancer has been observed over recent years. Like FOBT, a large-scale randomized study of flexible sigmoidoscopy has been performed, i.e., the Medical Research

Council once-only flexible sigmoidoscopy trial (with approximately 42 000 patients screened and twice as many controls), making it the largest randomized trial in gastroenterology. The baseline findings from this study have been published and the effects of flexible sigmoidoscopy and polypectomy on the incidence and subsequent mortality from colorectal cancer is anticipated in 2008 [9,10]. No such trials exist for total colonoscopy.

Barium enema

Barium enema has long been promoted by radiologists as an appropriate screening test for colorectal cancer. It is relatively cheap, can be performed by technicians, and is safe. However, the last few years have seen evidence accumulating that suggests that sensitivity for both significant adenomas and early cancers is just not high enough when compared to competing tests. In particular, the US national polyp study found sensitivity for adenomas 1 cm or larger to be only 48% in 862 paired enema and colonoscopic examinations performed in 580 patients [11]. There are no randomized trials of barium enema that aim to demonstrate an effect on disease-specific mortality from colorectal cancer, and such trials seem vanishingly unlikely in a climate where the palpable lack of enthusiasm on the part of radiologists to interpret the study and a general decline in the skills needed to do so in any event [12] are combined with overwhelming evidence in favor of competing techniques. It is hard to see how the barium enema could play a major part in any screening program at the present time or in the future, although the UK screening program pitches the test as an alternative when colonoscopy has been incomplete in those individuals whose FOBT is positive.

CT colonography (virtual colonoscopy)

The radiological community has embraced CT colonography (CTC) enthusiastically as a screening test for colorectal cancer. The test has been single-handedly responsible for considerable resurgence in interest in colorectal screening by radiologists, and it is worthwhile focusing much of this chapter on why this has happened and the corresponding evidence base.

On the face of it, CTC seems to combine the ideal attributes for a screening test for colorectal cancer – it appears sensitive, specific, safe, and acceptable. This section will attempt to pitch CTC as a screening test for colorectal cancer against the alternatives by considering the following prerequisites: Does it offer the chance of prevention or merely detect invasive cancer? Does it have appropriate sensitivity and specificity? Is it acceptable? Is it safe? Is it readily available? Is it cost-effective (i.e., cheap)? Are the results generalisable? Is it effective in reducing the disease-specific mortality from colorectal cancer?

Cancer prevention or cancer cure?

The point has been made already that in order for a screening test to potentially prevent cancer, it must be able to detect adenomatous polyps reliably. At the time of writing, there is little doubt that CTC can image polyps with great precision. The combination of helical CT scanning of the cleansed and distended colorectum with advanced 3D image rendering that simulated the colonoscopist's perspective (Figure 3.1) was first described in 1994 [13]. This abstracted work provided proof-of-principle – that CT could detect colon polyps by "virtual colonoscopy" – and precipitated a rash of studies that essentially used very similar methodology: the findings from CTC were compared with same-day, subsequent, intra-individual colonoscopy. In order to both facilitate recruitment and increase the prevalence of abnormality, practically all studies investigated symptomatic subjects who were scheduled for colonoscopy in any event. The landmark example of such a study was performed by Fenlon and co-workers who performed CTC and compared the findings with same-day colonoscopy in 100 subjects at high risk of colorectal

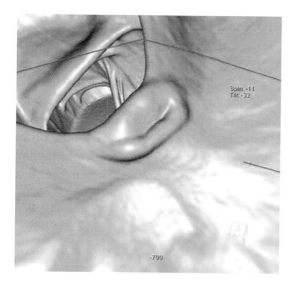

Figure 3.1 Endoluminal 3D perspective rendered image from a CT colonography examination. The examination has reached the cecum and a normal ileocecal valve is shown.

neoplasia [14]. The radiologists interpreting the CTC examinations detected 20 (91%) of the 22 polyps measuring 1 cm or larger, 46 of 51 (91%) adenomas measuring 6 mm or larger, and all 3 cancers [14]. From the many, many very similar that studies have followed, there is no doubt from their combined results that CTC has the potential to image polyps with high sensitivity, offering the potential for cancer prevention rather than cure alone. There is considerable continuing debate, however, as to with what facility CTC detects polyps overall, with some studies finding it equivalent to colonoscopy [15] while others have found it no better than barium enema [16]. This debate is considered in the following section. It should also be borne in mind that CTC cannot determine with certainty the histology of most polyps it depicts and, as a result, most studies have concentrated on "polyp" detection – i.e., all polyps are considered, which includes hyperplastic varieties for example. Hyperplastic polyps are generally believed to carry no potential for malignant transformation.

Test characteristics: sensitivity and specificity

Meta-analysis is appropriate when trying to reconcile divergent results from different studies: it allows us to derive an overall point-estimate of diagnostic performance by mathematical synthesis of the results of a number of individual studies. There have been at least three attempts to meta-analyze studies of CTC [17,18,19]. The most recently published was sponsored by the European Society of Gastrointestinal and Abdominal Radiology (ESGAR) and European Association of Radiology (EAR), and meta-analysed data from 24 component studies with 4181 participants [17]. The investigators found high per-patient average sensitivity of 93% (95% CI: 73% to 98%) and average specificity of 97% (95% CI: 95% to 99%) for CTC when used to detect polyps 1 cm or larger [17]. Test characteristics declined when smaller polyps were included in the analysis, with per-patient average sensitivity of 86% (95% CI: 75% to 93%) and average specificity of 86% (95% CI: 76% to 93%) when the diagnostic threshold was lowered to include patients whose polyps were 6 mm or larger (Figure 3.2). Declining detection of smaller polyps is a consistent finding in practically all comparative studies of CTC. Cancers are generally larger than polyps and, as such, should be the easiest lesions to detect. The ESGAR meta-analysis found that 144 of 150 cancers were detected by CTC, with an overall detection rate of 96% (95% CI: 91% to 99%).

The other two meta-analyses similarly found CTC to have high sensitivity and specificity [18,19]. However, perhaps the most interesting finding was that they did

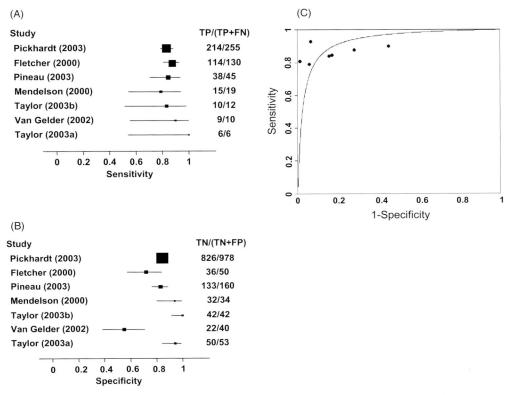

Figure 3.2 **Per-patient meta-analysis for detection by CT colonography of polyps measuring 6 mm or larger (taken from reference [17]). Meta-analysis was based on data from 1834 patients in seven studies, 477 of which were identified with one or more medium or large polyps. From this model, the operating point has an average sensitivity of 86% (95% CI: 75% to 93%; range 79% to 100%) and specificity of 86% (95% CI: 76% to 93%; range 55.0% to 100%). (A) Forest plot of sensitivity; (B) Forest plot of sensitivity; (C) ROC plot of sensitivity vs 1-specificity.**

not report any problems with data extraction. In contrast, the authors of the ESGAR meta-analysis reported very considerable difficulty with obtaining the requisite data from component studies, and considered the poor quality of data reporting to be the major finding from their review [17]. For example, the authors found that they were able to extract a fully populated 2×2 contingency table for per-patient data (for any polyp size category) from the information presented in the published article in only 50% of the component studies; data were available for a further 5 only after contacting the corresponding author [17]. In the context of screening for colorectal cancer, test characteristics for per-patient performance are the central statistic because the patient is the unit of assessment, not the polyp. This is because it matters not whether the patient has one or many polyps; once a polyp of a size sufficient to precipitate subsequent colonoscopy has been identified, colonoscopy will be scheduled in all cases. In contrast, the authors of the ESGAR meta-analysis found that a 1×2 contingency table for per-polyp data (for any polyp size category) could be extracted from all component studies [17].

This focus on per-polyp detection has not helped the cause of CTC when the data is assessed independently by health policymakers. For example, investigators have usually chosen to ignore data clustering and have not accounted for it in their analyses. Data clustering is an inevitable consequence of per-polyp analyses because some patients will have more than one polyp. In an extreme example, imagine a study of 10 patients, 9 of whom have a single polyp each but where the tenth patient has 10 polyps (i.e., the study population has 19 polyps in total). That single patient will contribute disproportionately to a per-polyp analysis. If the single polyp in all other patients is detected but none are detected in the tenth patient (because of poor bowel preparation or distension, for example), then sensitivity will be 0.47 (i.e., 9 of 19 polyps detected). Per-patient analysis of the same data will yield very different results, a sensitivity of 0.9 (i.e., 9 of 10 patients correctly categorized). It is important to recognize that when a single polyp is well depicted in a patient, other polyps in the same patient are also likely to be well depicted because they are all subject to similar circumstances of bowel preparation, distension, colonic anatomy, compliance with breathing instructions, etc. The converse is also true. This interdependence of data (also known as "clustering" or "correlation") is frequently ignored.

It was also clear to the ESGAR meta-analysts that polyp matching was a prime source of uncertainty when attempting to evaluate the results of component studies, and again there was a lack of clarity with how this data was handled by authors. Because patients can have more than one polyp, it is necessary to match the polyps depicted by CTC with those detected (or not) by subsequent colono-scopy in order to arrive at sensible estimates of sensitivity and specificity. Polyps can be different sizes and located at different sites in the colon and so matching algorithms have been based on polyp size and location, with endoscopy invariably used as the reference standard. However, it is unclear how successful these match-ing algorithms are in reality. For example, when asked to locate the tip of their instrument, endoscopists frequently cannot do this with precision [20]. Furthermore, endoscopic estimates of polyp size are frequently inaccurate [21]. The result is that the reference test is unreliable and this will impact negatively on any assessment of CTC. Also, it is now clear that the impact of such matching schemes is more damaging than suspected initially [17,22]. For example, if there is disagreement between CTC and colonoscopy regarding the size of a polyp then the result will be both a false-negative and false-positive score for CTC because the polyp detected by colonoscopy was not depicted by CTC (= false-negative), and the polyp depicted by CTC did not match the polyp detected by colonoscopy (= false-positive).

The net result is that the point estimates arrived at by meta-analysis must be regarded with a degree of suspicion because the methodology and quality of data-reporting in component studies is questionable. This is discussed further in the section on "generalizability" below.

Acceptability

It is well understood that any screening test has to be acceptable to screenees or compliance will likely suffer as a result. Although the data are relatively immature, there are a number of pointers that indicate CTC is acceptable to patients. Van Gelder and colleagues assessed patient experiences and preferences both directly after CTC and subsequent colonoscopy, and 5 weeks later [23]. They found that patients experienced significantly less discomfort during CTC and that 71% of 249 patients preferred CTC directly after the procedures. However, this fell to 61% at 5 weeks, at which point whether a polyp was found or not emerged as a preference for colonoscopy. The authors concluded that while patients prefer CTC, the fact that considerations regarding outcome supplant temporary inconvenience in time should not be ignored [23]. Taylor and colleagues similarly investigated the experiences of patients having both barium enema and CTC, finding that patients suffered significantly less physical discomfort during CTC and were more satisfied with the procedure overall [24]. Later follow-up revealed that patients were significantly less prepared to undergo barium enema again and all of the patients expressing a preference for future examination indicated CTC [24]. Taylor and colleagues also investigated the experiences of 186 subjects undergoing CTC followed by flexible sigmoidoscopy or colonoscopy [25]. Again, the investigators found that CTC was significantly less uncomfortable than endoscopy, better tolerated, and was the preferred follow-up investigation of those expressing a preference [25]. However, they did find that patients were significantly more "satisfied" with endoscopy. This finding almost certainly relates to the environment in which the test is performed; during endoscopy, the patient is in very close proximity to the endoscopist and nurse, and there is plenty of opportunity for discourse (assuming sedation is not excessive). In contrast, CTC is performed in a relatively frightening environment with the patients lying alone on a "cancer-scanner," with the medical participants secreted safely in another room behind protective glass. Other workers have also found that CTC is well perceived when compared to colonoscopy [26].

Edwards and colleagues invited asymptomatic subjects for screening CTC, which was followed by colonoscopy if abnormal, and used a visual analog scale to determine acceptability [27]. Only 28.4% of eligible screenees attended but CTC was highly acceptable to participants, with most finding the experience better than expected [27].

Safety

Much has been made of the fact that CTC is safe, with several authors suggesting that there is no risk of perforation for example. However, hard data concerning adverse events is starting to emerge that suggests CTC does indeed carry a risk of significant adverse events (Figure 3.3). What is important is not whether there is a risk or not (it would be churlish to deny there is), but to determine exactly what this risk is and how it sits with competing tests in the context of a screening program.

Outside of the context of isolated case reports, the first authors to suggest that CTC does carry a risk of perforation were Sosna and co-workers, who presented abstracted data describing 9 perforations in 24 365 examinations, a perforation rate of 0.04% [28]. This work attracted negative criticism but the authors are to be congratulated for attempting to tackle a difficult subject in the face of those champions of the technique who have vested interests in its favorable portrayal. However, a valid criticism was that the data was obtained by questioning inter-nationally visible experts. This approach introduces selection and spectrum bias because only data from "visible" groups is collected. Supporting this, there is evidence that colonoscopy-associated adverse events are more frequent in non-expert/non-academic centres, than when experienced practitioners in "expert" centres are questioned [7]. In an attempt to circumvent this bias, Burling and colleagues performed a national survey of the United Kingdom, collecting data from all National Health Service hospitals [29]. They assembled data on 17 067 procedures from 50 centres: 13 patients (0.08%) suffered a potentially serious adverse event attributable to CTC, 9 of which were perforations. Four perforations were entirely asymptomatic, to give a symptomatic perforation rate of 0.03% (1 in

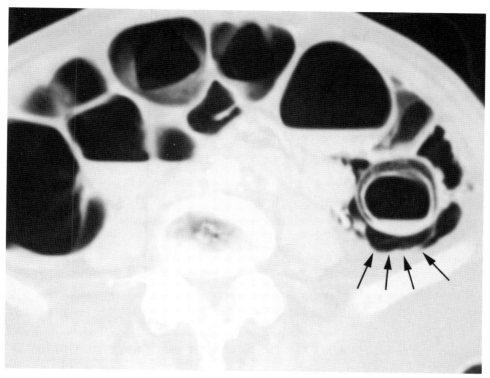

Figure 3.3 Axial 2D image from a CT colonography examination where colonic perforation had occurred inadvertently. There is extraluminal gas (arrows) surrounding the descending colon.

3413 patients). One patient required laparotomy but there were no deaths. The authors made the point that CTC is exquisitely sensitive to extra-colonic gas whereas this would go undetected by colonoscopy if the patient remained asymptomatic, and suggested that the germane comparison was the symptomatic perforation rate from CTC to the symptomatic perforation rate at colonoscopy, i.e., 0.03% versus 0.13% [29].

The same authors also investigated the degree of cardiovascular compromise experienced by patients undergoing both CTC and colonoscopy, since it is believed that cardiovascular depression as a consequence of sedation is a significant cause of serious adverse events during colonoscopy [30]. Using a Holter monitor to record cardiovascular events before, during, and after the procedures the authors were able to show that CTC was associated only with a mild tachycardia related to administration of intravenous spasmolytic whereas colonoscopy was associated with potentially serious cardiac arrhythmias and cardiovascular depression owing to the sedation that is inevitable in most patients if the procedure is to be comfortable [30]. It is also worth bearing in mind that the colonoscopists in this study were of high expertise and unlikely to represent the average practitioner, who may be inclined to administer more sedation when the "going gets tough."

Availability and cost-effectiveness

There is very little good-quality evidence regarding the availability of CTC and even less to inform decisions relating to cost-effectiveness. It is worth bearing in mind that 75% of the Earth's population have no access to CT scanning at all! There is, rightly, a general perception that access to CT scanners is both restricted and costly. Access will depend both on the local health care environment and the nature of the referral in question – e.g., self-referral for screening or clinician referral for investigation of the symptoms of colorectal cancer.

In a national survey of the United Kingdom, Burling and colleagues found that CTC was available in about one-third of National Health Service hospitals [31]. CTC was performed almost exclusively to investigate older patients with symptoms possibly indicating colorectal cancer, because this is the group perceived most at risk from adverse events related to colonoscopy, and diagnostic colonoscopy services are stretched to capacity [31]. Kalish and co-workers attempted to clarify current patterns and trends of CTC when used for screening, and investigated self-referral body imaging centres, identified via Internet advertising [32]. They identified 161 centres versus 88 identified in 2001, indicating expansion of this type of provision. However, immediate localities were wealthier, had higher levels of college education, and higher household income than the national average [32]. The authors concluded that while access to CTC was broadening, it was far from comprehensive. The bottom line from these studies and others is that access to CTC is relatively restricted at the time of writing.

Sonnenberg and colleagues were the first to attempt to determine the cost-effectiveness of using CTC to screen for colorectal cancer [33]. Using a Markov model, they concluded that screening by CTC would cost $24 586 per life-year saved, compared with $20 930 for colonoscopy. Furthermore, the authors concluded that colonoscopy remained more cost-effective than CTC even if the sensitivity and specificity of the latter rose to 100%. For the two screening procedures to become similarly cost-effective, the authors calculated that CTC needed an initial compliance rate up to 20% better than colonoscopy [33]. While many opinion-leaders have suggested that CTC is likely to be associated with improved compliance over and above colonoscopy, good-quality data proving this is conspicuous by its absence. Similarly, Heitman and co-workers also performed an economic evaluation, using decision analysis, to compare CTC with colonoscopy for colorectal cancer screening in patients over 50 years of age [34]. They calculated that CTC would cost $2.27 million extra per 100 000 patients screened; 3.78 perforation-related deaths would be avoided, but 4.11 extra deaths would occur from missed adenomas [34].

The glaring problem with such studies is that their models are populated with data obtained from the published literature, and their results therefore turn on the accuracy of these data. For all of the reasons rehearsed in the sections above, it would be difficult to decide what test characteristics to input for CTC, or indeed colonoscopy. For example, the sensitivity for polyps in the reasonable-quality CTC literature ranges between 45% and 97% [17]. If modeling the accuracy of CTC for screening, only a single study is available to submit data that reflects directly the population being investigated by the simulation [15]. As a result, it is now well established that the optimal approach to such modeling studies is to devise and execute a well-designed study to obtain the requisite data necessary to populate all relevant fields of the model. As a result, the model is populated with quality data that reflects real-world performance and costs rather than speculative assumptions. The results of the study can then be extrapolated beyond the confines of the study, via the model, with a reasonable chance of that the findings are evidence-based and believable. However, a central problem is that randomization is usually required in order to obtain the cleanest and most reliable data, and this methodology requires very large studies for the results to have reasonable statistical power. Also, because the data will be extrapolated, a higher statistical power than the conventional 80% is often required, especially when trying to model the effects on disease-specific mortality. At the time of writing, the author is aware of a single randomized study of CTC – the SIGGAR study [35] – and, even then, this study does not examine CTC in a screening situation.

Are results generalizable?

The sections above have described high per-patient average sensitivity and specificity for CTC, derived from meta-analysis. The fact remains, though, that these results have been arrived at by synthesis of studies performed by researchers in expert centres. How generalizable are these findings to day-to-day clinical practice?

It should be remembered that one meta-analysis could find only 24 studies whose methodology was acceptable enough to be included – there were 1398 potential candidates [17]. The prevalence of abnormality in the 24 studies selected ranged from 15% to 72% [17], clearly indicating that the patients examined must be from widely different populations. Emphasizing this, the ESGAR investigators found that when their meta-analysis was extended to include all polyps irrespective of size, the data from component studies was too heterogenous in both sensitivity (individual range 45% to 97%) and specificity (individual range 26% to 97%) for meaningful meta-analysis [17]. Such findings question the believability of the individual studies and must inevitably limit the generalizability of the results of meta-analysis. This is in complete contrast to the data from individual randomized trials of FOBT screening, which demonstrate no such heterogeneity when their results are combined [4]. Furthermore, only a single study of CTC has been performed on individuals genuinely representative of a group of asymptomatic screenees, and using technology representative of current best practice [15]. Some key opinion-leaders may quite rightly point out that this is the sum total of our evidence that CTC is suitable for colorectal cancer screening.

One study concluded that CTC was not yet ready for generalized implementation [36], but some of the investigators in that study had personal experience of only 10 patients. The statement is therefore no less ridiculous than suggesting that colonoscopy is not ready for generalized implementation because practitioners are not proficient after 10 colonoscopies (or mammograms in the case of mammographic screening). While the author would agree CTC is not yet ready for generalized implementation for colorectal cancer screening, this opinion is based on the fact that the results from many different studies are so disparate. This can only be explained by inherent biases, either toward CTC or colonoscopy, both overt and covert. Indeed, it has been noted that the results of studies of CTC seem to vary with the specialty of the principal investigator, faring well when studies are led by radiologists and poorly when led by gastroenterologists [37]. At best, the data from meta-analysis indicates the potential level of performance achievable for CTC, given good practice and implementation. At the same time, heterogeneity of data from component studies reflects the fact that the test is not yet ready for implementation on a wide scale.

Why might the results from different investigators be so variable? The FOBT studies are all in accord but in that case the result of the test is pretty simple to determine – the sample is either positive for blood or not, and the sample is read by a machine. The situation for CTC is very different because the result is contingent

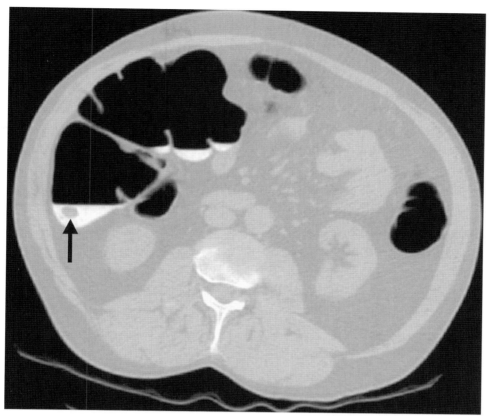

Figure 3.4 Axial 2D image from a CT colonography examination. Data displayed in this way is interrogated by scrolling through sequential images. 3D rendering may be used for problem-solving uncertain findings. In this case, positive oral contrast medium has been used to tag residual fluid and so distinguish it from potential lesions. There is a 10 mm cecal polyp (arrow) submerged in the tagged fluid.

on several factors and authors have debated which of these underpins discrepant trial results. Much has been made of the software used to display the CT imaging, namely whether the data is displayed as 2D transverse images (Figure 3.4) or as 3D endoluminal views (Figure 3.5). There is no doubt whatsoever that the 3D display used for the inauguration of "virtual colonoscopy" was responsible for most of its immediate appeal [13]. However, it rapidly became clear that the computer power necessary for such rendering was prohibitive in day-to-day clinical practice, and researchers rapidly adopted the much less computer- and time-intensive 2D transverse image approach to interpretation. At the time of writing, however, 3D analysis is no longer problematic because computational capabilities are no

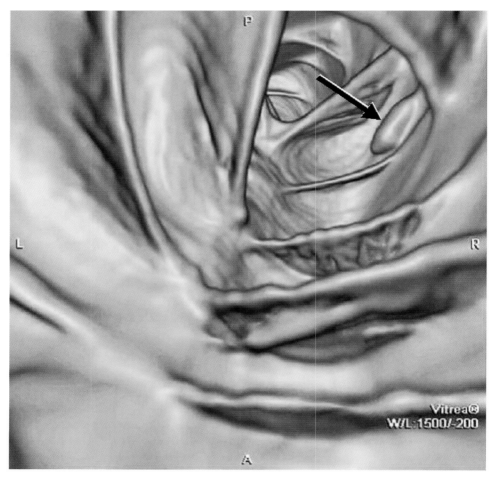

Figure 3.5   Endoluminal 3D perspective rendered image from a CT colonography examination. There is a 10 mm polyp seen in the distance (arrow).

longer the limiting factor in the critical path. Outstanding results have been obtained by research groups using both imaging paradigms so this is unlikely to be the major factor underpinning discrepant study results, although it may have brought considerable influence to bear in some studies. The same probably applies to other oft-implicated factors such as CT collimation and the quality of bowel preparation and distension (which is unlikely to be universally bad or good in most studies).

The author believes that it is the experience and training of the interpreting radiologist that is the major factor at the root of discrepant results. CTC is a novel technology and many investigators have acquired it and immediately implemented an "audit" of its performance via comparison with same-day colonoscopy. Many published studies merely represent initial experience with the technique and the published results incorporate the learning curve for the observers concerned. As already noted, one oft-cited multicentre study required CT observers only to have experience of 10 studies before their participation [36]. Unsurprisingly, the observers that had most a-priori experience fared best [37]. Contrast that methodology with the results from large multicentre studies of endoscopy, which show that polyp detection by practitioners continues to improve over many hundreds of examinations [38]. In the author's opinion, the question of whether CTC is generalizable will only be answered by large multicentre studies, incorporating many different radiologists, all of whom have reached a certain level of competence before they are assessed – the ACRIN2 study is one such example and its results are eagerly awaited [39].

In the meantime, what evidence do we have for the variability and level of individual observer performance? Several small studies have investigated this topic. A study of three observers before and after a period of directed training found that prior experience of gastrointestinal radiology conveyed an advantage but, surprisingly, the performance of one observer declined following training [40]. This observation is counter-intuitive and may reflect over-confidence following training, but nonetheless emphasizes the fact that competence cannot be assumed. A European multicentre study compared the interpretative performance of experienced CTC researchers with that of radiologists and radiographic technicians who had been trained using 50 endoscopically validated cases (a figure often suggested as adequate for training) [41]. Overall, 28 observers read 1084 examinations. Experienced observers detected more lesions overall (66% versus 51% for radiologists and 47% for technologists), and were significantly more accurate as well; 74.2% versus 66.6% for radiologists and 63.2% for technologists [41]. Interestingly, there was no significant difference between the trained radiologists and technologists but the best performing of these individuals reached the mean performance achieved by experienced observers. Similarly, some experienced observers fell below the median standard achieved by the other two groups. The take-home message, unsurprisingly, is that experienced observers perform best and that their level of performance cannot be achieved after 50 cases on average – the fact remains that individual performance is variable, irrespective of background. Other multireader studies have similarly found that prior experience enhances performance [42].

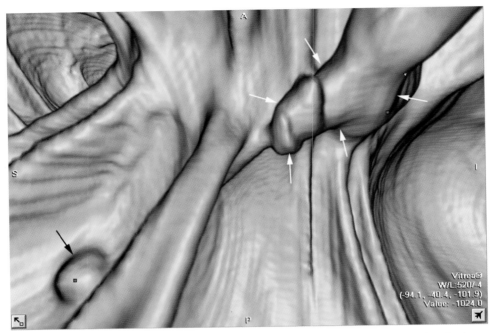

Figure 3.6   Perspective-rendered 3D endoluminal image showing a cancer (white arrows) and polyp (black arrow). The small squares placed on the polyps are CAD prompts, indicating the possible location of a polyp to the observer.

Computer-assisted-detection (CAD) systems have recently become widely available in the commercial marketplace after several years gestation in research laboratories. The hope is that by labeling polyps with visual prompts, less experienced readers will be able to detect polyps reliably (Figure 3.6). Those who interpret CTC currently will be well aware that it is crushingly tedious and time-consuming when compared to conventional abdomino-pelvic CT, and it is often suggested that CAD systems will accelerate interpretation, making it more time-efficient and less tedious [43]. The vast majority of studies of CAD have determined its performance in isolation – i.e., the CAD algorithm is applied to CTC studies where the location of polyps is known and its sensitivity and specificity is determined. The largest study to use this approach was performed by Summers and colleagues who found that CAD detected 89.3% of polyps 10 mm or larger in a test set of 792 patients [44]. The potential benefit of CAD assistance has been inferred indirectly by comparing the sensitivity of CAD and radiologists when asked to interpret the same dataset: Taylor and co-workers found that CAD was more sensitive than any of three experienced observers [45]. However, such studies assume that the observer will react accordingly to a true-positive CAD prompt. In reality, there is no guarantee that this will be the case. In a study of 10 readers who interpreted a dataset of 107 CTC studies both with and without CAD assistance, observers repeatedly chose to ignore true-positive prompts [46]. The reasons underlying this phenomenon are unclear but the author believes that much of this apparently illogical behavior can be abolished by a period of training. However, CAD significantly improved sensitivity overall; on average, 12 more polyps were detected by each reader when using CAD [46]. Also, interpretation time decreased significantly; by a mean of 1.9 minutes per patient for those with polyps and by 2.9 minutes for those without [46]. Other studies have also found that observers using a primary 2D analysis and CAD are as sensitive as those using a primary 3D read, while being faster [47]. The author believes that CAD will help the generalizability of CTC ultimately, but is insufficient to achieve this in isolation.

Effect on disease-specific mortality

There is no evidence whatsoever that CTC is able to reduce disease-specific mortality in the context of screening for colorectal cancer. However, it is not alone in this respect. Randomized evidence is available only for FOBT at the time of writing, where there is no doubt that its administration reduces deaths from colorectal cancer [1,2,3,4]. There has been a large randomized trial of screening by flexible sigmoidoscopy, but the effects on disease-specific mortality will not be available until 2008 [10]. The problem with disease-specific mortality as an endpoint is that huge trials are required because the index event (i.e., death by colorectal cancer) is relatively infrequent. The result is that tens of thousands of patients must be recruited in order to detect a difference reliably. Not only does this mean that such trials are time-consuming and very expensive, but there is a very considerable delay between the close of recruitment and analysis since cancer takes many years to develop and declare itself. In the meantime, good case-control studies exist that provide indirect evidence that polypectomy reduces the incidence of subsequent cancer [48,49]. It is on this type of study that the success of CTC (and colonoscopy) is predicated; if polypectomy reduces cancer, and CTC is good at detecting polyps, then it must follow that CTC can prevent cancer. This approach is not as evidence-based as a randomized controlled trial, but such trials seem vanishingly unlikely at the present time.

The author is aware of a randomized controlled trial of CTC – the UK SIGGAR trial – but this trial focuses on diagnosis of symptomatic cancer by CTC, barium enema, and colonoscopy, and is powered to detect differences in cancer detection rates (which in itself requires thousands of patients) [35]. Any differences in disease-specific mortality would require hundreds of thousands of patients to detect, and this type of information can only realistically be obtained by extrapolated models populated by trial data. The trial is not concerned with screening.

Summary

Summarizing the sections above, there is no doubt that colorectal cancer is an ideal candidate for screening, and there is excellent evidence (primarily from FOBT studies) that mortality can be reduced effectively. At the time of writing, CTC holds considerable promise as a viable screening procedure. This is because it seems safe, is acceptable to patients, and its potential performance is very good. However, there are serious doubts concerning its immediate generalizability although these can likely be overcome by training and by careful and considered dissemination of the test. More than a single, good study on asymptomatic screenees is also needed badly. There is a conspicuous absence of good data relating to cost-effectiveness and to the precise level of enhanced compliance it brings (if any) over and above alternative tests. More data on these topics are needed urgently if health policy-makers are to adopt CTC enthusiastically.

At the present time, CTC is probably viable as a screening tool where there is access to the technology and, most importantly, the requisite expertise for competent reporting. Although the vast majority of studies investigating CTC have made comparisons with colonoscopy, in many ways a more germane comparison is with the barium enema. Both are relatively safe, can be performed by technicians, and examine the whole colon. Barium enema has failed essentially because its sensitivity for target lesions, both adenomas and cancer, is just not good enough. This is probably not because of any intrinsic technical deficiency. Rather, it is because competent interpretation could not be achieved in a generalized setting, combined with little momentum to improve matters in the face of improving endoscopic services. CTC has provided radiologists with an unexpected second opportunity to capture the flag. However, if we allow CTC to disseminate in an uncontrolled and unregulated fashion, then it will ultimately suffer the same fate as the barium enema as a screening test. Alternatively, it could be argued sensibly that CTC is best pitched as a diagnostic test for patients with symptoms of colorectal cancer (of whom there are many), and to abandon ambitions of large-scale screening altogether.

REFERENCES

1. Hardcastle, J. D., Chamberlain, J. O., Robinson, M. H., *et al.* Randomised controlled trial of faecal-occult-blood screening for colorectal cancer. *Lancet*, **348** (1996), 1472–7.
2. Kronborg, O., Fenger, C., Olsen, J., Jorgensen, O., and Sondergaard, O. Randomised study of screening for colorectal cancer with faecal-occult-blood test. *Lancet*, **348** (1996), 1467–71.
3. Mandell, J. S., Bond, J. H., Church, T. R., *et al.* Reducing mortality from colorectal cancer by screening for faecal occult blood: Minnesota colon cancer control study. *N Engl J Med*, **328** (1993), 1365–71.
4. Towler, B., Irwig, L., Glasziou, P., *et al.* A systematic review of the effects of screening for colorectal cancer using the faecal occult blood test, hemoccult. *BMJ*, **317** (1998), 559–65.
5. Patz, E. F., Goodman, P. C., and Bepler, G. Screening for lung cancer. *N Engl J Med*, **343**:22 (2000), 1627–33.
6. Raffle, A. E. Honesty about new screening programmes is best policy. *BMJ*, **320** (2000), 872.
7. Bowles, C. J., Leicester, R., Romaya, C., *et al.* A prospective study of colonoscopy practice in the UK today: are we adequately prepared for national colorectal cancer screening tomorrow? *Gut*, **53** (2004), 277–83.
8. Garvican, L. Planning for a possible national colorectal cancer screening programme. *J Med Screen*, **5** (1998), 187–94.
9. Atkin, W. S., Cuzick, J., Northover, J. M., and Whynes, D. K. Prevention of colorectal cancer by once-only sigmoidoscopy. *Lancet*, **341** (1993), 736–40.
10. UK flexible sigmoidoscopy screening trial investigators. Single flexible sigmoidoscopy screening to prevent colorectal cancer: baseline findings of a UK multicentre randomised trial. *Lancet*, **359** (2002), 1291–300.
11. Winawer, S., *et al.* National polyp study: a comparison of colonoscopy and double contrast barium enema for surveillance after polypectomy. *N Engl J Med*, **324** (2000), 1766–72.
12. Halligan, S., Marshall, M., Taylor, S. A., *et al.* Observer variation in the detection of colorectal neoplasia on double contrast barium enema: implications for colorectal cancer screening and training. *Clin Radiol*, **58** (2003), 948–54.
13. Vining, D. J., Gelfand, D. W., Bechtold, R. E., *et al.* Technical feasibility of colon imaging with helical CT and virtual reality. *Am J Roentgenol*, **162**:suppl. (1994), 104.
14. Fenlon, H. M., Nunes, D. P., Schroy, P. C. 3rd, *et al.* A comparison of virtual and conventional colonoscopy for the detection of colorectal polyps. *N Engl J Med*, **341** (1999), 1496–503.
15. Pickhardt, P. J., Choi, J. R., Hwang, I., *et al.* Computed tomographic virtual colonoscopy to screen for colorectal neoplasia in asymptomatic adults. *N Engl J Med*, **349** (2003), 2191–200.
16. Rockey, D. C., Paulson, E., Niedzwiecki, D., *et al.* Analysis of air contrast barium enema, computed tomographic colonography, and colonoscopy: prospective comparison. *Lancet*, **365** (2005), 305–11.
17. Halligan, S., Altman, D. G., Taylor, S. A., *et al.* CT colonography in the detection of colorectal polyps and cancer: systematic review, meta-analysis, and proposed minimum data set for study level reporting. *Radiology*, **237** (2005), 893–904.

18. Mulhall, B. P., Veerappan, G. R., and Jackson, J. L. Meta-analysis: computed tomographic colonography. *Ann Intern Med*, **142** (2005), 635–50.

19. Sosna, J., Morrin, M. M., Kruskal, J. B., *et al.* CT colonography of colorectal polyps: a meta-analysis. *Am J Roentgenol*, **181** (2003), 1593–8.

20. Shah, S. G., Saunders, B. P., Brooker, J. C., and Williams, C. B. Magnetic imaging of colonoscopy: an audit of looping, accuracy and ancillary manoeuvres. *Gastrointest Endosc*, **52** (2000), 1–8.

21. Gopalswamy, N., Shenoy, V. N., Choudhry, U., *et al.* Is in vivo measurement of size of polyps during colonoscopy accurate? *Gastrointest Endosc*, **46** (1997), 497–502.

22. Halligan, S. Causes of false-negative findings at CT colonography. *Radiology*, **238** (2006), 1075–7.

23. van Gelder, R. E., Birnie, E., Florie, J., *et al.* CT colonography and colonoscopy: assessment of patient preference in a 5-week follow-up study. *Radiology*, **233** (2004), 328–37.

24. Taylor, S. A., Halligan, S., Burling, D., Marshall, M., and Bartram, C. I. Intra-individual comparison of patient acceptability of multidetector-row CT colonography and double contrast barium enema. *Clin Radiol*, **60** (2005), 207–14.

25. Taylor, S. A., Halligan, S., Saunders, B. P., *et al.* Acceptance by patients of multidetector CT colonography compared with barium enema examinations, flexible sigmoidoscopy, and colonoscopy. *AJR*, **181** (2003), 913–21.

26. Svensson, M. H., Svensson, E., Lasson, A., and Hellstrom, M. Patient acceptance of CT colonography and conventional colonoscopy: prospective comparative study in patients with or suspected of having colorectal disease. *Radiology*, **222** (2002), 337–45.

27. Edwards, J. T., Mendelson, R. M., Fritschi, L., *et al.* Colorectal neoplasia screening with CT colonography in average-risk asymptomatic subjects: community-based study. *Radiology*, **230** (2004), 459–64.

28. Sosna, J., Blachar, A., Amitai, M., and Bar-ziv, J. Assessment of the risk of perforation at CT colonography (abstr). *Eur Radiol*, **15**:suppl. 3 (2005), 16.

29. Burling, D., Halligan, S., Slater, A., Noakes, M., and Taylor, S. A. Potentially serious adverse events associated with CT colonography performed in symptomatic patients: a survey of the United Kingdom. *Radiology*, **239** (2006), 464–71.

30. Taylor, S. A., Halligan, S., O'Donnell, C., *et al.* Cardiovascular effects at multi-detector row CT colonography compared with those at conventional endoscopy of the colon. *Radiology*, **229** (2003), 782–90.

31. Burling, D., Halligan, S., Taylor, S. A., Usiskin, S., and Bartram, C. I. CT colonography practice in the United Kingdom: a national survey. *Clin Radiol*, **59** (2004), 39–43.

32. Kalish, G. M., Bhargavan, M., Sunshine, J. H., and Forman, H. P. Self-referred whole-body imaging: where are we now? *Radiology*, **233** (2004), 353–8.

33. Sonnenberg, A., Delco, F., and Bauerfeind, P. Is virtual colonoscopy a cost-effective option to screen for colorectal cancer? *Am J Gastroenterol*, **94** (1999), 2268–74.

34. Heitman, S. J., Manns, B. J., Hilsden, R. J., *et al.* Cost-effectiveness of computerized tomographic colonography versus colonoscopy for colorectal cancer screening. *CMAJ*, **173** (2005), 877–81.

35. http://www.ncchta.org/projectdata/1_project_record_notpublished.asp?PjtId=1366&SearchText =colonography. Accessed May 25, 2006.

36. Cotton, P. B., Durkalski, V. L., Pineau, B. C., *et al*. Computed tomographic colonography (virtual colonoscopy): a multicentre comparison with standard colonoscopy for detection of colorectal neoplasia. *JAMA*, **291** (2004), 1713–19.

37. Halligan, S. and Atkin, W. A. Unbiased studies are needed before virtual colonoscopy can be dismissed. *Lancet*, **365** (2005), 275–6.

38. Atkin, W., Rogers, P., Cardwell, C., *et al*. Wide variation in adenoma detection rates at screening flexible sigmoidoscopy. *Gastroenterology*, **126** (2004), 1247–56.

39. http://www.acrin.org/6664_brochure.html. Accessed May 25, 2006.

40. Taylor, S. A., Halligan, S., Burling, D., *et al*. CT colonography: effect of experience and training on reader performance. *Eur Radiol*, **14** (2004), 1025–33.

41. ESGAR ESGAR CT colonography study group investigators. Effect of directed training on reader performance for CT colonography: multi-centre study. *Radiology*, **242** (2007), 152–61.

42. Johnson, C. D., Toledano, A. Y., Herman, B. A. *et al*. Computerized tomographic colonography: performance evaluation in a retrospective multicentre setting. *Gastroenterology*, **125** (2003), 688–95.

43. Bond, J. H. Progress in refining virtual colonoscopy for colorectal cancer screening. *Gastroenterology*, **129** (2005), 2103–6.

44. Summers, R. M., Yao, J., Pickhardt, P., *et al*. Computed tomographic virtual colonoscopy computer-aided polyp detection in a screening population. *Gastroenterology*, **129** (2005), 1832–44.

45. Taylor, S. A., Halligan, S., Burling, D., *et al*. Computer-assisted reader software versus expert reviewers for polyp detection on CT colonography. *AJR*, **186** (2006), 696–702.

46. Halligan, S., Altman, D., Mallett, S., *et al*. CT colonography: multi-reader multi-case (MRMC) assessment of performance with and without computer assisted detection. *Gastroenterology*, **131** (2006), 1690–9.

47. Taylor, S. A., Halligan, S., Slater, A., *et al*. Polyp detection using CT colonography: primary 3D endoluminal analysis versus primary 2D transverse analysis with computer-assisted reader software. *Radiology*, **239** (2006), 759–67.

48. Atkin, W. S., Morson, B. C., and Cuzick, J. Long-term risk of colorectal cancer after excision of rectosigmoid adenomas. *N Engl J Med*, **326** (1992), 658–62.

49. Selby, J. V., Friedman, G. D., Ouesenberry, C. P., and Weiss, N. S. A case-control study of screening sigmoidoscopy and mortality from colorectal cancer. *N Engl J Med*, **326** (1992), 653–7.

4

The surgical approach to colorectal cancer

Ian R. Daniels and Richard J. Heald

Introduction

The traditional approach to surgery for colorectal cancer was to remove the segment of bowel containing the tumor and then assess the specimen by pathological analysis. This, together with the surgeon's assessment for metastatic disease during the operation, led to the patient's tumor being "staged." The traditional staging system for rectal cancer was the Dukes' Stage, described in 1937 by the pathologist Cuthbert Dukes and related to the degree of invasion of the tumor through the bowel wall, and the presence or absence of involved local lymph nodes [1,2]. This system was later used for all colorectal cancers and allowed a prognosis to be given to the patient. Later developments in staging led to other systems, such as those of Jass and Astler-Coller, and the current system of the AJCC, namely TNM [3,4,5,6]. However, these systems are based solely on tumor invasion and nodes, yet there are many other factors that are associated with local recurrence or the development of distant metastases. These include tumor differentiation, mucin production, vascular invasion, peritoneal invasion and in rectal cancer, involvement of the circumferential resection margin (CRM) [7]. With the introduction and development of radiological techniques to stage the tumor prior to surgery and the introduction of preoperative therapies to downsize/downstage the tumor, the importance of optimal surgical resection has increased.

In this chapter, we will be discussing the techniques involved with the surgical approaches to rectal cancer, and how the information from the radiological assessment may influence the operative decisions, together with the recognition that the principles of surgery for rectal cancer can be applied to colon cancer.

Historical basis for surgery for colorectal cancer

Bubo (the owl) is an apostem breeding within the anus in the rectum with great hardness but little aching. This I say, before it ulcerates, is nothing else than a hidden cancer, that may not in the beginning of it be known by the site of the eye, for it is all hidden within the rectum; and therefore it is called bubo, for as bubo, i.e., an owl, is always dwelling in hiding so that this sickness lurks within the rectum in the beginning, but after passage of time it ulcerates, and eroding out of the anus, comes out. And often it erodes and wastes all of the circumference of it so that . . . it may never be cured with man's cure. But if it pleases God, that made man out of nothing, to help with this unspeakable virtue; which forsooth, is known thus: the leech put his finger into the anus a thing as hard as stone, sometimes only on one side only, sometimes on both, so that it permits the patient to have egetion, it is bubo (cancer) for certain. Signs, forsooth, of ulceration are these: the patient cannot abstain from going to the privy because of aching and pricking and that twice or thrice within one hour; and he passes a stinking discharge mixed with watery blood. (John of Ardenne (fourteenth century))

There is nothing new in the principles of managing rectal cancer. John of Ardenne recognized the symptoms of rectal cancer, the signs of rectal cancer, but also recognized that the relationship of the circumferential component of the tumor was the key determinant and that circumferential involvement was associated with incurable disease. Six centuries later, the symptoms have not changed, the importance of circumferential involvement is the key determinant, and early recognition of the condition could lead to cure. But during those six hundred years, the developments in surgery have led the way with the improvement of outcome of rectal cancer.

Morgagni (AD 1689–1771) was the first to propose an operation for cancer of the rectum, and Fajet performed the first attempt at resection of the rectum for an inflammatory lesion in 1739. The first recorded suggestion for enterostomy or colostomy was made by Littré (1658–1726), as reported by Fontanelle in 1710. During the first half of the nineteenth century, the operation gained popularity, with Freer, a surgeon in Birmingham, performing the first in England in 1815. Whilst Fajet attempted the first rectal resection, it was Jacques Lisfranc (1790–1847) who carried out the first successful perineal or posterior resection in 1826. But it was not until the end of the nineteenth century that the operation for cancer of the rectum was performed at all frequently [8]. From the turn of the nineteenth century, procedures for rectal carcinoma were classified as follows:
(1) Perineal excision
(2) Perineal resection

(3) Resection through the vagina
(4) Combined abdominal and perineal excision
     The abdomino-anal operation
     The radical abdominoperineal operation
     The perineo-abdominal operation

Following the introduction of anesthesia and the acceptance of anti-sepsis, proce-
dures for rectal cancer became more common. After the pioneering work of Lisfranc,
the perineal excision continued to be carried out by European surgeons such as
Theodore Billroth. However, this method fell into disuse and remained so until
Verneuil revived it in 1873 and suggested that coccygectomy, originally described by
Amussat, would facilitate the extirpiration by providing extra room [9].

    Vincent Czerny in 1883, finding that he could not complete a resection of the
rectum by the perineal route, turned the patient over and completed the resection
through the abdomen; thus, introducing the abdominoperineal excision. The English
surgeon, W. Ernest Miles, who whilst a House-Surgeon under Allingham at St. Marks
reported the first series of abdominoperineal excisions (Miles procedure) [10],
recognized that cancer of the rectum may spread in any of three distinct ways:

(1) by direct extension through continuity of tissue,
(2) by way of the venous system,
(3) by means of the lymphatic system.

In 1939, whilst Miles was publishing his book *Rectal Surgery: A Practical Guide to
the Modern Treatment of Surgical Disease* [11], Dixon, in America, described the
sphincter-preserving anterior resection. Although previously alluded to by
Moynehan in the UK, it was Dixon who described the first large series. He
performed the operation in three stages, initially by defunctioning the rectum
with a colostomy, then by an anterior resection with the colostomy remaining,
before closure of the colostomy [12,13]. During the later part of the twentieth
century, refinements of the surgical technique led to an improvement in survival,
principally through a reduction in surgical morbidity; but the major problem
facing surgeons who performed rectal resection was the subsequent development
of local recurrence within the pelvis. This often led to fistulation into the bladder or
other viscera, sciatic nerve involvement, or invasion into local bony structures;
and once present, there was a $< 5\%$ five-year survival. Indeed, the series reported
from 1940 to 1980 in the surgical literature report local recurrence rates from 10%
to 49% [14,15]. The identification that the cause of local recurrence was the
incomplete removal of the rectum and its draining lymphatics contained within
the mesorectum was the key determinant in improving surgical outcome [16]. This,

in parallel with the recognition of the pathologically assessed circumferential resection margin, led to the dramatic fall in local recurrence rates that have been seen following the acceptance of the principle of total mesorectal excision (TME) [17]. The key feature of this surgical principle is the identification of the plane of cleavage along which surgical resection must be performed. This has become recognized as the "Holy Plane" (of Heald) [18].

The embryological basis of surgical technique

The principles of colorectal surgery are based upon an understanding of the embryological origins of the section of bowel to be removed. The theory behind TME is that cancer spread will tend, initially at least, to remain within the embryological hindgut "envelope" – the mesorectum. Although the gut developed partly outside the abdomen, when it returned, it retained its lympho-vascular integrity although now being attached by a series of peritoneal folds. The bowel remains separate from the other organs by a collagenous areolar tissue that surgically forms a "plane that can be cleaved at operation" and is almost entirely avascular. In performing a TME, it is the dissection along this perimesorectal avascular plane around the midline hindgut into the depths of the pelvis that led to an improvement in local recurrence rates. Straying into the field of cancer spread is a common cause of involved surgical margins and residual pelvic disease, whilst straying out can damage the autonomic nerve layers and is a common cause of impotence.

Surgical planes: the interaction with radiology

The key determinant for the successful treatment of rectal cancer is the recognition of the importance of the mesorectal fascia and the relationship of the tumor to it by all members of the multidisciplinary team (MDT). The presence of tumor at the mesorectal fascia is associated with a high rate of local recurrence and poor survival. The optimal surgical procedure for rectal cancer is the complete removal of the mesorectum contained within the fascia and the delivery of a specimen with the fascia intact. This is the first interaction with radiology. The radiologist can supply the MDT with information on the tumor position within the rectum, its depth of spread within the mesorectum, its relationship to the surrounding organs, its relationship to the anal sphincter, and the presence of other adverse factors, such as involved lymph nodes or vessels; all of which allow improvements in planning the operation – for being well equiped is being safe.

The technique of total mesorectal excision

The original idea for TME was born from the practice of surgery. The mesorectum only becomes a reality if each individual surgeon performs a meticulous operation delivering to the histopathologist a specimen that allows accurate comparison to the preoperative imaging. The recognition of the individual planes allows the MDT to stage the tumor accurately and provides the "road-map for treatment" (Figure 4.3).

Of the fascial layers, the innermost "Holy Plane" is that which surrounds the midline hindgut within its lymphovascular envelope – the core. The surrounding layers form a neural layer and a Wolffian ridge layer that develop from the paired structures outside the hindgut. The Japanese have adopted this idea and compared the pelvic anatomy with the layers of an onion.

The "Holy Plane" is around the integral visceral mesentery of the hindgut – the mesorectum, which is a complete fatty and lymphovascular surround on all aspects in the middle third of the rectum. In the upper third, the anterior aspect is covered only by the peritoneum with "mesorectum" at the back and enveloping the sides as the peritoneal reflection tapers forward toward the "cul de sac." In the lower third of the rectum, virtually no fatty tissue intervenes between the anterior aspect of the rectum and the back of the prostate. At its upper extremity, the prostate has an important fascial attachment to the lowest extremity of the shiny front surface fascia of the encircling mid-rectal mesorectum. The surgeon has to divide this layer to enter the plane between the rectum and the prostate. In the female, the middle third has a rather thin and tenuous fatty layer between the rectum and vagina with Denonvillier's Fascia being difficult to identify [19]. Posteriorly and postero-laterally, the plane is well defined around the globular expanding bi-lobed mesorectum. A condensation of the fascia called the "recto-sacral ligament" often presents a barrier to the surgeon below the promontory.

The TME concept can be seen to fit within the six-step MDT process:
(1) High-resolution body-coil MRI for local rectal staging combined with CT staging of chest, abdomen, and pelvis for distant disease
(2) MDT meeting, case discussion, and treatment planning
(3) Selective preoperative therapy on the basis of preoperative MRI staging
(4) Precision surgery – TME for cancers of the mid/low rectum, "TME minus" or partial ME for upper 1/3 cancers, or enhanced abdominoperineal excision for low/ano-rectal cancers.
(5) Histopathological macroscopic/microscopic specimen assessment.

(6) MDT assessment and decision regarding postoperative therapy.

TME for the surgeon comprises 6 basic principles:

(1) Perimesorectal "Holy Plane" dissection under direct vision with three-directional traction.

(2) Specimen-orientated surgery and histopathology, of which the object is an intact mesorectum with no tearing of the surface and no CRM involvement.

(3) Quirke-style histopathological audit for CRM involvement as the principal immediate outcome measure.

(4) Preservation of the autonomic plexuses and nerves, on which sexual and bladder function depend

(5) Reconstruction of the rectum using a colonic pouch and therefore a reduction in the number of permanent colostomies

(6) Stapled low pelvic reconstruction, usually using the Moran triple stapling technique plus creation of a short colon pouch anastomosed to low rectum or anal canal.

The important steps in performing a TME

1. The incision – A long midline incision from the symphysis pubis to within a few centimeters of the xiphisternum.
2. Manual palpation and inspection – Laparotomy
3. Packing – Careful packing and retraction of the intestines upward and to the right is crucial to provide clear access to the pelvis.
4. The pedicle package – Identification of the plane between the back of the inferior mesenteric vessels and the gonadal vessels, ureter, and preaortic sympathetic nerves (Figure 4.1).
5. The high ligations – The inferior mesenteric artery is divided 1–2 cm anterior to the aorta. The inferior mesenteric vein is divided above its last tributary close to the pancreas. The ascending left colic artery and either the accompanying inferior mesenteric vein or its last tributary from the left colon may also need to be divided separately to complete the vascular isolation of the specimen with full mobilization for ultra low pouch anastomosis (Figure 4.2).
6. The division of convenience – Division of the sigmoid mesentery and sigmoid colon well above the cancer. This facilitates the opening of the perimesorectal planes (Figure 4.3).

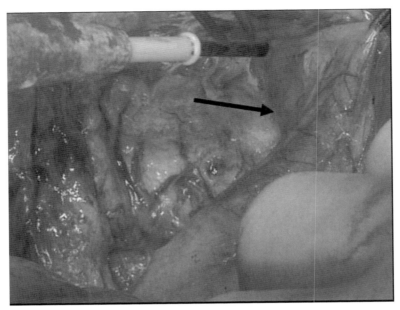

Figure 4.1   The pedicle package – the mesorectal fascia covering the inferior mesenteric artery and vein.

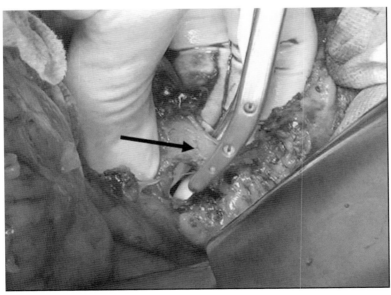

Figure 4.2   The high ligation of the inferior mesenteric artery using a Ligasure Ultrasonic scalpel™.

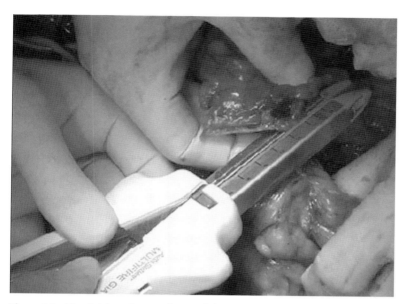

Figure 4.3 The division of convenience of the sigmoid colon using a transverse intestinal stapler.

7. The pelvic dissection – Initially, the surgical dissection is performed poster-iorly. Forward traction demonstrates the shiny posterior surface of mesorec-tum within the bifurcation of the superior hypogastric plexus (Figure 4.4). The plane is extended downward toward and beyond the tip of the coccyx (Figure 4.5).

8. Division of the recto-sacral ligament or fascia – This condensation may constitute an apparent barrier to downward progress requiring positive divi-sion with scissors or diathermy.

9. Lateral pelvic dissection – Forward dissection of the "Holy Plane" around to the sides, gently easing the adherent hypogastric nerves off the mesorectal surface under direct vision.

10. The so-called "lateral ligaments" – Laterally, the inferior hypogastric plexus is adherent to the mesorectum, and the overlying fascia forms a condensation that allows branches of the nerves to enter the mesorectum. Dissection in this area will give the impression of a "lateral ligament" that previously was ligated and divided (Figure 4.6). This almost certainly was a division of the inferior hypogastric plexus formed from the sympathetic hypogastric nerves coming from above and the "erigent" parasympathetic nerves, formed from the roots of the sacral plexus (S2, S3, S4), coming forward to it from behind (Figure 4.7).

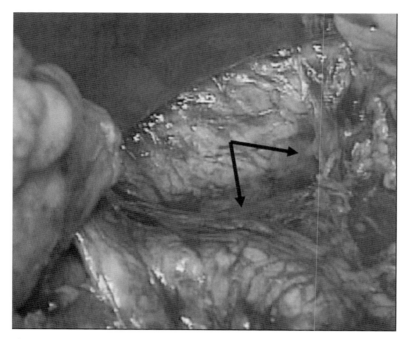

Figure 4.4   The "wishbone" shape of the diverging superior hypogastric nerves.

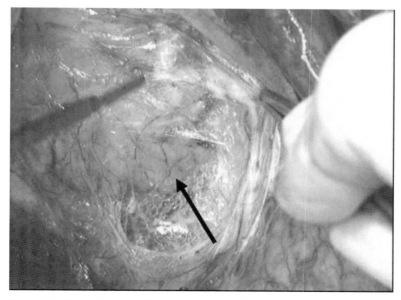

Figure 4.5   Dissection through the loose areolar tissue between the sacral fascia and the posterior mesorectum.

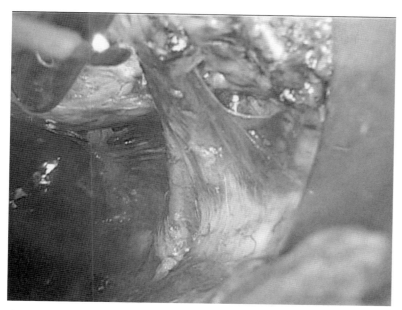

Figure 4.6   The erigent pillars can be seen outside the parietal fascia with the fascia tented against the rectum forming the "lateral ligaments."

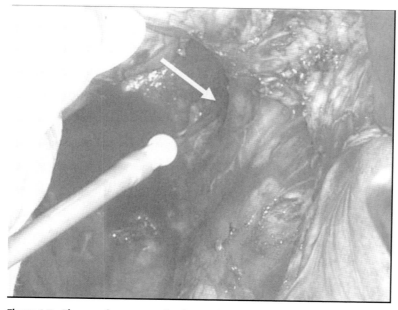

Figure 4.7   The sacral nerves coming forward and forming the inferior hypogastric plexus.

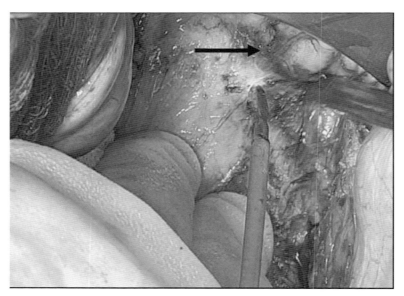

Figure 4.8   The anterior dissection showing Denonvillier's Fascia (white layer) and the plane between it and the vesicles (black arrow) and prostate.

Another often-described structure that is only rarely seen is the middle rectal artery. Anatomical studies have now confirmed that this occurs only rarely. Anteriorly and antero-laterally, the plane of dissection encompasses the peritoneal reflection that forms a positive identification of the backs of the seminal vesicles. Anterior retraction of these facilitates the development of the areolar space between the vesicles and the smooth front of the mesorectal specimen – this fascia is called Denonvillier's Fascia (Figure 4.8). Inferiorly, this has to be divided as it is adherent to the posterior capsule of the prostate. At this point, it is important to avoid damage to the neurovascular bundles (of Walsh) that constitute the distal condensation of the inferior hypogastric plexuses.

11. Rectal division – After complete mobilization of the rectum down to the pelvic floor, the rectum is divided by a cross-stapler. This divides and closes the distal rectum and ano-rectal remnant and allows reconstruction with either a straight-stapled anastomosis or creation of a colonic J-pouch and then anastomosis.

12. Delivery of the specimen – the complete mesorectal block containing the tumor, mesorectum and covered by the mesorectal fascia is seen (Figures 4.9 and 4.10).

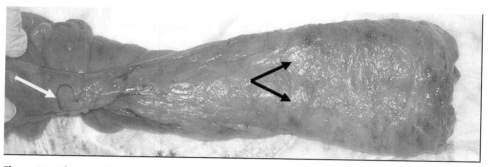

Figure 4.9   The posterior mesorectum forming a bi-lobed (black arrows) and the origin of the inferior rectal artery (white arrow).

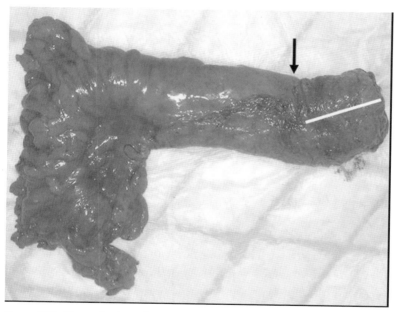

Figure 4.10   The excised specimen showing the peritoneal reflection (black arrow) with the distal rectum surrounded by the mesorectum (white line) and the distal sigmoid colon.

Optimal surgical technique

The delivery of an optimal specimen has been the basis for many years of the training workshops held at the North Hampshire Hospital and the Pelican Cancer Foundation. Indeed, international acceptance of the principles of TME and the workshop-directed live surgery have resulted in significant improvements in the outcome for rectal cancer in many countries. The Swedes were the first to institute a training program that has resulted in a reduction in the number of surgeons operating on rectal cancer and increasing specialization. Data from the follow-up of those patients treated, following the introduction of the program, has shown a reduction in CRM involvement, a low ($< 5\%$) rate of local recurrence and an increased number of sphincter-saving operations. This project formed the basis of the Pelican–Trent–Macmillan project that targeted improved multidisciplinary care and expanded the disciplines involved in this project. This project included the introduction of MRI training for radiologists and attempts to standardize the delivery of oncological therapy. It also built on the standardization of histopathological staging through the increased use of macroscopic grading of specimens – a system that has now been adopted for national use. The UK National Health Service adopted this project and delivered through The Pelican Cancer Foundation the English National MDT–TME Development Course that has rolled out a program of Colorectal MDT Development.

Laparoscopic surgery

The laparoscopic approach to colorectal cancer surgery has developed over the last ten years and it has been introduced into many hospitals in the UK. There is now a body of evidence, some from randomized laparoscopic colorectal cancer trials that demonstrate equivalent oncological results to open surgery, but with a reduction in morbidity, reduced blood loss, and reduction in length of hospital stay. However, apart from the randomized study from the UK (CLASICC), these trials excluded rectal cancer [20]. In rectal cancer, it is accepted that laparoscopic rectal cancer surgery is more challenging than laparoscopic colon cancer surgery, but over the next few years with the development of improved instrumentation there will be an increased use in rectal cancer. However, laparoscopic surgery will not fully replace open surgery but improved selection of patients will mean that the laparoscopic approach is another weapon in the armamentarium against cancer.

Colon cancer: the next challenge

With the improvement in outcome from rectal cancer, the difference in survival between rectal and colon cancer has narrowed with a greater improvement in rectal than colonic. This may be reflected in the improved staging in rectal cancer and the selection of locally advanced disease for a preoperative strategy, although this may also be related to an improvement in rectal cancer surgery. The challenge though for the next decade is to develop improved staging in colon cancer and possibly introduce preoperative therapy.

Conclusion

The revolution in multidisciplinary care has been the recognition that preoperative therapy gives better results than postoperative in terms of reducing local recurrence and improving survival. However, the use of preoperative therapy is associated with side effects and ideally patients should be selected as those in whom the benefit will be greatest. To achieve this requires accurate preoperative staging and comparison of the excised specimen to the staging. For this to occur, patients selected for surgery must receive optimal surgical care delivered through meticulous attention to technique. The demonstration of the benefit of TME and the delivery of a complete surgical specimen has dramatically improved outcome in rectal cancer through a reduction in local recurrence. This attention to detail must now be carried forward into colon cancer, where outcome is being reported to be worse than rectal cancer for the first time. We expect to see further improvements in staging colon cancer and potentially the use of preoperative therapy; with these we must see optimal surgical technique – the next challenge.

REFERENCES

1. Dukes, C. E. The classification of cancer of the rectum. *J Pathol Bacteriol* **35** (1932), 323–31.
2. Dukes, C. E. Histological grading of rectal cancer. *Proc Royal Soc Med* **30** (1937), 371–6.
3. Astler, V. B. and Coller, F. A. The prognostic significance of direct extension of carcinoma of the colon and rectum. *Ann Surg*, **139** (1954), 846–52.
4. Jass, J. R., Atkin, W. S., *et al.* The grading of rectal cancer: histological perspectives and multivariate analysis of 447 cases. *Histopathology*, **10** (1986), 437–59.
5. Jass, J. R., Love, S. B., *et al.* A new prognostic classification of rectal cancer. *Lancet*, **1** (1987), 1303–6.
6. Fleming, I., Cooper, J., *et al. AJCC Cancer Staging Manual* (Philadelphia. Lippincott-Raven, 1997).
7. Quirke, P., Dixon, M. F., *et al.* Local recurrence of rectal adenocarcinoma due to inadequate surgical resection. *Lancet*, **ii** (1986), 996–9.
8. Cromer, C. D. The evolution of the colostomy. *Dis Colon and Rectum*, **22** (1968), 256–80.
9. Amussat, J.-Z. *Memoire sur la possibilite d'etablir an anus artificiel dans la region lombaire sans penetrer dans le peritoine* (Paris: Lu a L'Academie Royale de Medicine, 1839).

10. Miles, W. E. A method of performing abdomino-perineal excision for carcinoma of the rectum and terminal portion of the pelvic colon. *Lancet*, **35** (1908), 320–1.

11. Miles, W. E. *Rectal Surgery: A Practical Guide to the Modern Surgical Treatment of Rectal Diseases* (London: Cassell and Company Ltd., 1939).

12. Moynihan, B. G. A. The surgical treatment of cancer of the sigmoid flexure and rectum. *Surg Gynaecol Obstet*, **6** (1908), 463–6.

13. Dixon, C. F. Surgical removal of lesions occuring in the sigmoid and rectosigmoid. *Am J Surg*, **46** (1939), 12–17.

14. Phillips, R. K. S., Hittinger, R., *et al.* Local recurrence following curative surgery for large bowel cancer in the rectum and recto-sigmoid. *Br J Surg*, **71** (1984), 17–20.

15. Pescatori, M., Mattana, C., *et al.* Outcome of colorectal cancer. *Br J Surg*, **74** (1987), 370–2.

16. Heald, R. J. and Husband, E. M. The mesorectum in rectal cancer surgery: the clue to pelvic recurrence? *Br J Surg*, **69** (1982), 613–16.

17. Heald, R. J., Moran, B. J., *et al.* The Basingstoke experience of total mesorectal excision 1978–1997. *Arch Surg*, **133** (1998), 894–9.

18. Heald, R. J. The "Holy Plane" of rectal cancer. *J Roy Soc Med* **81** (1988), 503–8.

19. Denonvillier's, C. Anatmie du périnée. *Bull et Mém Soc Anat* (Paris, 1836).

20. Guillou, P., Quirke, P., *et al.* Short-term endpoints of conventional versus laparoscopic-assisted surgery in patients with colorectal cancer (MRC CLASICC Trial) multicentre, randomised controlled trial. *Lancet*, **365** (2005), 1718–26.

5

Laparoscopic surgery

Anthony Antoniou and Ara Darzi

This chapter will examine the evidence for and against laparoscopic surgery in the field of colorectal carcinoma and summarize the exciting possibilities now available in the treatment of the disease.

Introduction

The first description of the use of laparoscopic surgery for colorectal resection for malignancy was in 1991 [1]. Twenty patients underwent laparoscope-assisted colon resection. Procedures undertaken included right hemicolectomy, sigmoid colectomy and a low anterior resection. Prior to this, laparoscopic surgery was already established, and even the norm, for the treatment of gallbladder disease and the surgical management of hiatus hernia. A great deal of skepticism and controversy surrounds the use of laparoscopic surgery for colorectal cancer resection following previous reports of port site metastases when the technique was applied in other specialties [2,3,4,5,6,7,8,9,10,11,12,13,14]. Surgeons have re-examined the role of laparoscopic surgery for many surgically treated malignancies, including colorectal carcinoma [15].

The potential advantages of laparoscopic surgery have been well documented, including decreased hospital stay, a reduction in postoperative pain, and a quicker return to normal function, together with less immune function disruption [16,17]. The attributes would be most beneficial to a cancer patient with studies showing a lower incidence of long-term complications and better quality of life in the first 12 months after surgery [18,19]. Despite the obvious benefits, only 1%–2% of all colorectal cancer resections in the UK are performed laparoscopically.

Laparoscopic colectomy: operative technique

Most colonic tumors are amenable to excision, unless they are fixed owing to local spread. The importance of adhering to sound oncological principles during laparoscopic surgery should never be forgotten. These include no-touch technique, en bloc resection of tumor, and involved structures together with oncological lymphadenectomy.

The inclusion of hand-assisted devices increases the accessibility for colorectal procedures [20]. A prospective randomized trial comparing hand-assisted and standard laparoscopic colectomy [21] showed that hand-assisted laparoscopic surgery retained all the benefits of the standard laparoscopic approach, with the convenience of a hand to aid during surgery. It also seems likely that the inclusion of a hand-assisted device reduces the rate of conversion to open when compared to a totally laparoscopic approach [22,23,24,25,26,27].

Potential advantages of the laparoscopic approach

Gastrointestinal motility

An obvious advantage of the laparoscopic approach for the cancer patient is the reduction in postoperative ileus. Early experience with laparoscopically assisted abdominoperineal resection confirmed that postoperative ileus was reduced as measured by the time to passage of flatus [28]. A combination of reduced postoperative pain [29,30,31,32,33] and a reduction in the handling of the bowel together with the use of a closed operative environment all contribute to early gastrointestinal recovery [34,35]. Various randomized trials have shown clear evidence of earlier return of bowel function with laparoscopic colectomies compared to open [36,37,38,39]. A recent study by Vignali *et al.* has shown that laparoscopic colectomy for cancer in octogenarians is safe and beneficial, including preservation of postoperative independence and reduction of length of hospital stay [40]. The latter study will broaden the boundaries for surgery in the elderly.

Quality of life

It is obvious that quality of life has many component parameters that can be measured and the majority of studies have focused on postoperative pain. As laparoscopic cases are often allowed to eat earlier than traditional cases, regular oral analgesia is often used, thereby causing an apparent decrease in the usage of parenteral analgesics. Randomized trials in which some of these variables are controlled have shown that there are definite benefits to postoperative pain in the laparoscopic group on day 1. However, in subsequent days, there are no significant differences in postoperative pain between laparoscopic and open groups [41]. Other studies have now confirmed less analgesic requirements in laparoscopic surgery compared with open surgery [35,37,39,41,42,43].

Length of hospital stay

One of the major potential economic advantages of laparoscopic surgery is to reduce hospital stay and thus decrease hospital costs. Many trials exist giving a wide variety of data. Both retrospective and prospective studies have shown ranges from 5 to 16 days in hospital [35,43,44,45,46,47]. Randomized trials in the main support the view that a laparoscopic-assisted colectomy results in a shorter time in hospital [29]. Recently, Nelson and colleagues reported on a larger group of patients and showed a definite significant decrease in hospital stay [42]. Other randomized trials have confirmed this [35,36,37,38,39,41,42,43].

Fast-track surgery/Enhanced recovery programs

Multimodal rehabilitation programs or fast-track surgery [48,49] have been applied after both laparoscopic [50,51] and open [52] colonic resections. Studies have shown a reduced hospital stay to about 2 or 3 days. A combined approach within the context of fast-tracking includes technical aspects such as minimally invasive (laparoscopic) surgery, anesthesiological aspects (short-acting anesthetics and regional anesthesia), and optimized postoperative pain relief with continuous epidural analgesia in major procedures, together with adjustment of general post-operative care principles with avoidance of nasogastric tubes, drains, and with early institution of oral feeding and mobilization [48,49,53,54]. Recent evidence suggests that the difference observed between laparoscopic and open surgery may be less significant when perioperative care is optimized within an enhanced recovery program. A recent study compared short-term outcomes of laparoscopic and open resection of colorectal cancer within such a program and despite perioperative optimization of open surgery, short-term outcomes were better following laparoscopic surgery. There was no deterioration in quality of life or increased cost associated with the laparoscopic approach [55].

Adequacy of excision and lymph node harvest

One of the initial major concerns of the laparoscopic approach for curative cancer resection was that it could lead to a breach of well-established oncological principles: inadequate resection margins, poor lymph node harvest, and port-site metastases to name a few. Since these early experiences, many studies have demonstrated adequate excision margins and lymph node harvest [56,57,58,59].

High ligation of the vascular pedicle provides oncological lymphadenectomy and reduces the likelihood of recurrence [60]. Corder and collaborators studied 143 consecutive patients and found no difference in recurrence nor mortality compared with the method of vascular ligation [61].

Long-term outcomes and survival evidence from trials

When evaluating laparoscopic surgery and comparing it with the open approach, complications, morbidity and mortality, oncological safety, and achievement of proposed benefits are the most important parameters to consider. In 1997, Bonjer *et al.* reviewed the literature regarding port-site metastases and found an incidence between 0% and 1.9% in the laparoscopic group, and between 0.8% and 3.3% in the open surgery group [62]. It therefore appears that the phenomenon of wound recurrence was not simply a laparoscopic problem.

Lacy and co-authors showed recurrence rates comparable with open surgery, and a low incidence of port-site metastases [63]. This trial acted as the precursor to larger, multicenter prospective randomized trials. The three main trials include: (1) The COLOR trial (Colon carcinoma Laparoscopic or Open Resection), a European muticenter randomized that began in 1997. The primary end point of the study is cancer-free survival after 3 years [64]. (2) The US-based NCCTG trial focused on disease-free survival, oncological resection, morbidity and mortality, and quality of life issues, as well as cost-effectiveness [65]. (3) The MRC-CLASICC trial, based in the UK, examined the adequacy of resection, and compared recurrence, morbidity and mortality rates, and disease-free survival to that of open surgery [66]. The study showed that laparoscopic-assisted surgery for cancer of the colon is as effective as open surgery in the short term and is likely to produce similar long-term outcomes. With the extension of the learning curve shown in the CLASICC trial, laparoscopic surgery for rectal cancer with careful selection using MRI may result in similar outcomes to those seen in laparoscopically assisted colon cancer surgery. The clinical outcomes of a surgical therapy study group compared

428 open colectomies and 435 laparoscopically assisted operations, and demonstrated clearly that recurrence and survival rates were similar in both groups. They found, however, a significant advantage for the laparoscopic group in analgesic requirement and length of stay [42]. Initial reports from these randomized trials are positive and point to laparoscopic surgery having a positive role in the management of colorectal malignancies in the future [19].

Patient selection

Patient selection plays a very important role in performing a successful laparoscopic procedure. Risks can be divided into general and specific.

General risks

It is important for the laparoscopist to understand possible complications and to have a fully informed discussion with the patient prior to surgery. The minimal access and surgical skills of laparoscopy impose limitations of patient selection, surgical procedure, and surgeons. Obesity, previous bowel surgery, inflammatory bowel disease, peritonitis following previous surgery, and two prior midline incisions may contribute to failure to achieve pneumoperitoneum and thus may contribute to bowel injury [67,68]. Patients must be forewarned of the procedure being converted to a laparotomy if problems arise. Open laparoscopy is not failsafe in achieving successful pneumoperitoneum or in preventing laparoscopic complications [69,70,71]. There may be intrinsic complications from a surgical-related disease process, regardless of whether the procedure was performed by laparoscopy or laparotomy. Obtaining an informed consent should include a discussion of the potential problems associated with the technique of laparoscopy. Anesthetic risks particular to laparoscopy result from the production of a pneumoperitoneum together with placing the patient in the Trendelenburg position. This may not only pose ventilation–perfusion challenges to the anesthetists but also alter intra-abdominal blood flow [72]. Laparoscopic instruments and equipment are more complex when compared to instruments used at laparotomy, and therefore more prone to failure. It is important that the public perception of minimal access surgery as "simple surgery" be balanced with a full discussion of the attendant risks.

Specific intra-operative risks

In surgical practice, complications may arise intra-operatively, immediately postoperatively, or much later. These complications may be related to anesthesia, bleeding, infection, or damage to structures adjacent to the surgical site. Laparoscopy is no exception. Some complications, however, are specific to laparoscopic surgery [68,69,73,74,75,76,77], including malfunction of equipment, trocar injuries, endoscopic surgical instrument injuries, and thermal injuries. Immediate management of laparoscopic complications will help minimize sequelae.

Principles of cancer surgery

The major principles of surgical resection of colon and rectal cancer are, first, removal of the entire cancer with enough bowel proximal and distal to the tumor mass to encompass the possibility that there has been submucosal lymphatic tumor spread and, secondly, removal of regional mesenteric draining lymphatics, so-called "lymphadenectomy." With the introduction of laparoscopic resections, there is a minimization of psychological and functional consequences of surgery without sacrificing any of the first two precepts. Thus, the right hemicolectomy, transverse colectomy, or left hemicolectomy are founded on anatomic structures, specifically the ileocolic, middle colic, and left colic arteries, defining what is both a convenient anatomic boundary for standard colonic resection and also providing for adequate regional lymph node clearance. There are recurring observations that stage-adjusted results are better in expert hands. These issues have become more important as the management of mesorectal, mesenteric, regional, and hepatic extension assumes a greater importance. Extra effort to achieve ideal margins is especially important in surgery for the low sigmoid colon and rectum. Short-cuts or technical inadequacies by the surgeon performing a limited resection likely will lead to inadequate proximal, distal, or radial margins, thus needlessly increasing the probability of regional recurrence.

Rectal cancer surgery

The surgical convention for rectal cancer has been changing steadily. Older standards dictated that any distally located adenocarcinoma of the rectum that could be palpated digitally required abdominoperineal (APR) resection. Recently, surgeons have been placing low anterior anastomoses closer and closer to the anal verge. The most extreme extension of this is the colo-anal anastomosis. One of the limiting factors in the surgical cure of patients with distal rectal carcinoma is the distal margin. A 2 to 2.5-cm margin distal to the tumor has been shown to help prevent submucosal lymphatic or isolated suture-line recurrence of rectal carcinomas. The most important limiting factor is the radial margins, particularly in males with low lying tumors. Ideally, the choice of operation should not make a difference in the surgeon's ability to achieve a satisfactory radial margin. Total mesorectal excision, as advocated by Professor Heald [78], has produced both increased long-term survival and, in particular, low incidence of local tumor recurrence, which indicates that this technique is mandatory for all tumors of the middle and lower third of the rectum.

The procedure

Prior to any form of laparoscopic surgery, especially involving left-sided surgery, the tumor is tattooed at endoscopy to allow visual identification of its position at laparoscopy.

Laparoscopic colorectal surgery is initiated in the supine position with the legs in the Lloyd-Davis position whether a right- or left-sided procedure is being undertaken (Figure 5.1). This will allow greater stability of the patient on the table when the latter is tilted. A urinary catheter is introduced, a nasogastric tube is inserted, and the abdomen is prepared in the usual fashion. The nurse is at the foot of the table with the surgeon standing on the side of the patient opposite the pathology being resected (Figure 5.2). Traditionally, in open surgery, the surgeon would

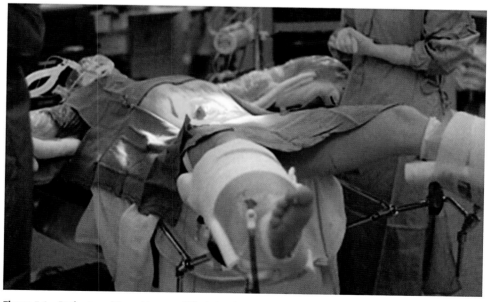

Figure 5.1 Patient positioned in a modified Lloyd–Davis position.

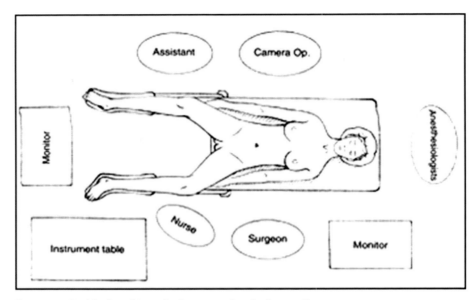

Figure 5.2   Positioning of team for laparoscopic colonic resection.

stand on the same side of the pathology being removed. A 10–12-mm port is introduced in the infraumbilical region via an open (Hassan) technique. Once the port is in position, a pneumoperitoneum is produced using carbon dioxide. This will allow the introduction of a camera into the peritoneal cavity and subsequent safe insertion of additional ports.

Once the camera is in position, the patient is placed in a steep Trendelenberg (head down) position and rotated away from the pathology to be resected. Further ports are inserted under direct vision to avoid any complications of insertion. The ports are positioned to allow manipulation of the bowel and to allow access to the vascular pedicle in question (Figures 5.3 and 5.4). Once the ports are in place, the small bowel is directed to the opposite side of the pathology and kept in position by altering the patient position by tilting the operating table. The next step is to isolate the main arterial supply to the segment of colon or rectum being removed.

Right hemicolectomy

The small bowel is placed in the left upper quadrant with adequate exposure being achieved once the duodenum is visualized. The ileocolic artery is identified by placing traction on the cecum and its origin isolated close to the duodenum. It can then be divided using an endoscopic stapling device. Dissection then proceeds from

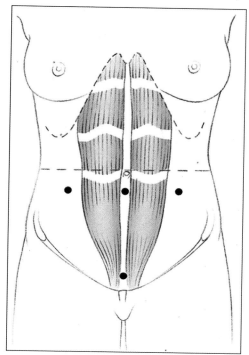

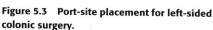

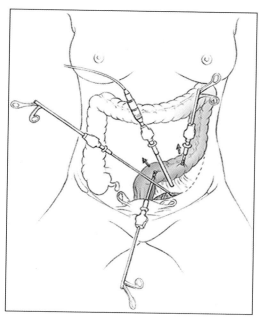

Figure 5.3   Port-site placement for left-sided colonic surgery.

Figure 5.4   Introduction of instruments for left-sided colonic surgery.

medial to lateral always staying above Toldt's fascia. Beneath this fascia, lie the ureter and the gonadal vessels and therefore provides a means to avoid damaging these vital structures. The mesentery is raised off the retroperitoneum and carried on to the hepatic flexure. This medial-to-lateral dissection differs from the conventional lateral to medial dissection in that of open surgery (Figure 5.5). The colon is then detached from its lateral connections to the abdominal wall and the terminal ileum mobilized. Finally, the greater omentum is removed from the transverse colon, and the right colon now becomes a midline structure. The next step involves making a small (5–6 cm) incision in the midline around the umbilicus to exteriorize the right colon and complete the right hemicolectomy (Figures 5.6 and 5.7).

Left hemicolectomy and anterior resection

The port-site placements are similar to that of a right hemicolectomy with some surgeons favoring a suprapubic port. The patient is placed in a deep Trendelenberg position with the patient dropped to the right. The sigmoid colon is placed under

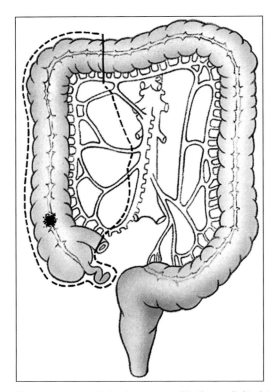

Figure 5.5   Boundaries incorporated in the medial to lateral dissection involved in a right hemicolectomy.

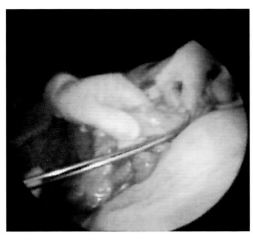

Figure 5.6   Exteriorization of the right colon in a right hemicolectomy.

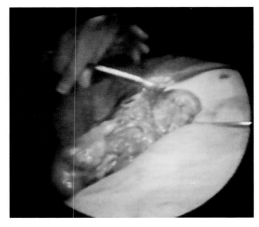

Figure 5.7   Returning the bowel into the abdominal cavity following resection and anastomosis.

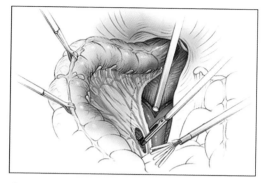

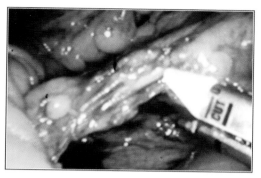

Figure 5.8 Medial to lateral dissection for a sigmoid colectomy/anterior resection with isolation of the inferior mesenteric artery.

Figure 5.9 Isolation of the inferior mesenteric artery.

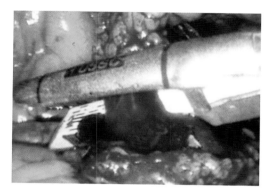

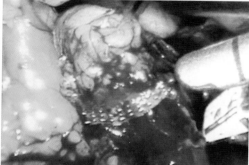

Figure 5.10 Staple ligation of the inferior mesenteric artery close to the aorta producing a "high tie."

traction and retracted to the left-hand side. The peritoneum at the rectosigmoid junction is incised allowing air to dissect under the peritoneum (Figure 5.8). The dissection is continued proximally until the origin of the inferior mesenteric artery is identified. The artery can be divided close to its origin from the aorta thus producing a "high tie" (Figures 5.9 and 5.10). Once again the mesentery to the left colon is elevated from the retroperitoneum, using blunt dissection, from medial to lateral. This dissection is continued up to the splenic flexure. In an anterior resection, a classic total mesorectal excision can be carried out laparoscopically, identifying a bloodless plane (Figure 5.11). Once again, the lateral dissection detaches the colon from its lateral attachments. As in open surgery, great care is taken to mobilize the splenic flexure to avoid damage to the spleen. The rectum can

(A)

(B)

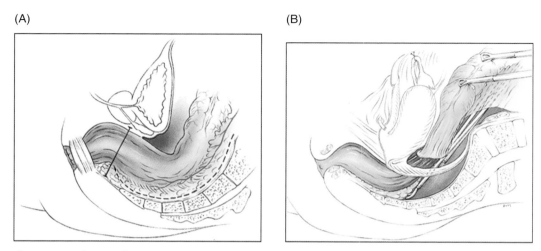

Figure 5.11   Diagramatic representation of a laparoscopic TME.

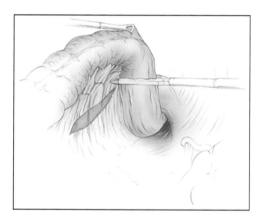

Figure 5.12   Transection of mobilized rectum.

be transected intra-abdominally (Figure 5.12) and exteriorized through a small left iliac fossa incision (Figure 5.13). Some surgeons prefer a Pfannensteil incision if further pelvic dissection is necessary. The colorectal anastomosis can still be performed using a CEEA stapling device with the anvil being positioned with the bowel exteriorized. The colon is then reintroduced into the abdomen, the wound closed and the pneumoperitoneum re-established. The colorectal anastomosis can then be achieved laparoscopically (Figures 5.14 and 5.15).

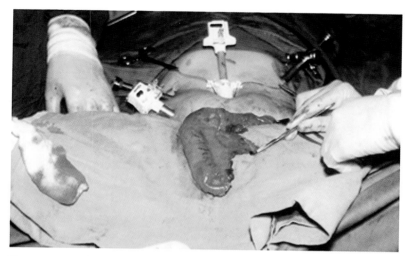

Figure 5.13   Delivery of specimen through a left iliac fossa incision.

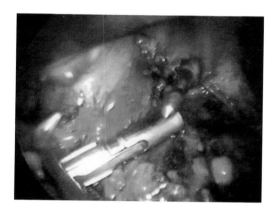

Figure 5.14   Intracorporeal stapled anastomosis.

The requirements for a successful anastomosis

Once the tumor has been excised, the two ends of bowel are joined together. This can be achieved either by using sutures or stapling devices. Every anastomosis requires

    a good blood supply to the two ends of the anastomosis
    accurate apposition to the two ends of the anastamosis be achieved
    that the two ends of the anastomosis be tension free
    that fecal contamination of the anastomosis be kept to a minimum.

The blood supply of the rectum is more precarious than that to the other parts of the gastrointestinal tract. With this in mind, middle and lower third

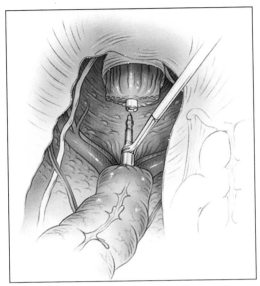

Figure 5.15   Diagramatic representation of an intracorporeal-stapled anastomosis.

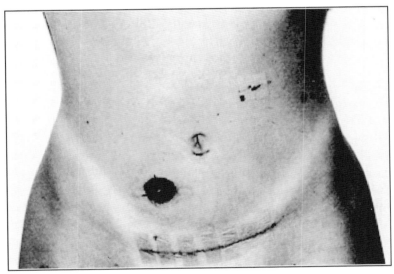

Figure 5.16   Defunctioning loop ileostomy following a laparoscopic low anterior resection.

rectal anastomoses are covered by a defunctioning loop ileostomy to allow the pelvic anastomosis to heal (Figure 5.16). The ileostomy is then reversed following a contrast study to check its integrity after 3 to 6 months (Figure 5.17).

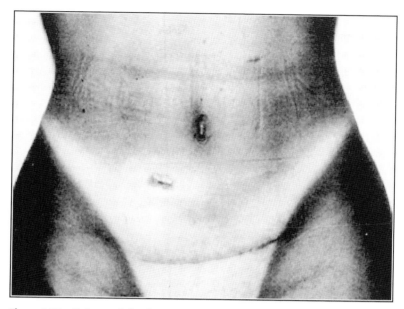

Figure 5.17   Abdomen following reversal of loop ileostomy for a laparoscopic low anterior resection.

Abdominoperineal excision of rectum

This procedure progresses exactly the same for an anterior resection with the total mesorectal excision being taken down to the pelvic floor. The perineal stage of the procedure is identical to that required for the conventional open approach (Figures 5.18 and 5.19). The extent of the pelvic dissection that remains to be completed from below will depend on the laparoscopic experience of the abdominal surgeon and the technical difficulty of the case.

Conversion from laparoscopic to open surgery

Initially in the learning curve of laparoscopic colorectal surgery there was a high conversion rate. This was only to be expected as this will always happen with the implementation of new technology and techniques to medicine. However, some surgeons continued to see high conversion rates and it was felt that this was probably because of inappropriate case selection. Identification of factors contraindicating laparoscopic surgery may well minimize inappropriate case selection. Certain factors have been identified as reasons for necessitating conversion to an open procedure. These are tumor fixity, either to adjacent organs or pelvic side wall/retroperitoneum,

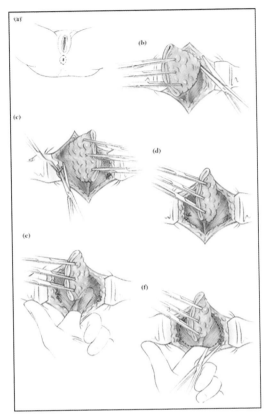

Figure 5.18   Superficial perineal dissection for an abdominoperineal resection.

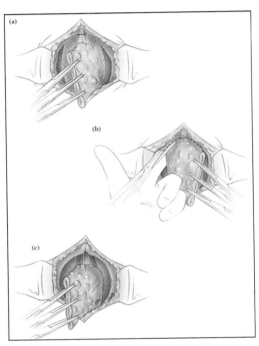

Figure 5.19   Deep perineal dissection for an abdominoperineal resection.

tumor not localized, mesenteric tumor spread, small bowel obscuring the operative field, obesity causing mesenteric bulking, and, finally, technical difficulties.

Port-site recurrences

When laparoscopic colorectal surgery was in its infancy, a disturbing phenomenon of port-site recurrence was observed, even for early Duke's A carcinomas. A number of studies have looked at port-site metastases [39,43,63]. These were randomized-controlled trials that showed no port-site metastases in patients over a follow-up period of between 7 and 46 months. This is consistent with other prospective studies in which the incidence of port-site metastases did not exceed

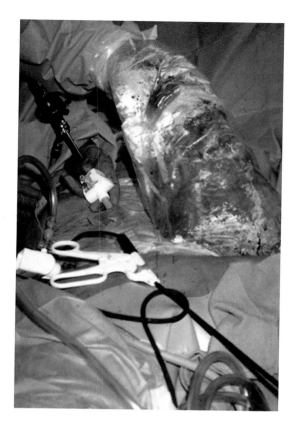

Figure 5.20   **The use of a wound protector to deliver the specimen.**

1.3% [79,80,81]. This lead to the opinion that the phenomenon of port-site metastases may be connected to the underlying tumor biology rather than to the technique of laparoscopy. A more meticulous approach to oncological principles such as minimal handling of the tumor, fixation of trocars to the abdominal wall, the use of wound protectors (Figure 5.20), and allowing the gas to discharge before removal of the trocars may well have contributed to the diminution of this phenomenon.

Summary

It is now emerging that laparoscopic colorectal resection for carcinoma is producing comparable results to those of open cancer surgery. Laparoscopic surgery is proving to be oncologically sound with regard to specimen resection, clearance, and lymph node harvest. It appears that the phenomenon of port-site metastases was because of poor operative technique together with learning curve issues, and that the technology at the same time also played a role. Reports from earlier non-randomized series are demonstrating a wound recurrence rate not dissimilar to that of open surgery, and it is fully expected that results from randomized trials will support this.

Continued experience with laparoscopic colectomy has demonstrated that morbidity and mortality levels are again similar to open surgery. However, the distinct advantages of less pain, less wound infection, improved cosmesis, and earlier return of intestinal motility are beyond doubt. Laparoscopic surgery for cancer resection has had a tough fight to gain a place in surgical practice and is demonstrating that it can deliver on its initial promise.

Summary tables comparing laparoscopic and open resections utilizing randomized-controlled trials

Randomized trials investigating return of bowel function after laparoscopic colectomy			
Number of trials	Total number of patients	Time to bowels open significantly shorter than open	References
4	212	Yes	[36],[37],[38],[39]

Randomized trials investigating reduction in pain after laparoscopic colectomy				
Number of trials	Total number of patients	Less pain	Significantly less pain	References
6	641	Yes	Yes	[35],[37],[39],[41],[42],[43]

Randomized trials investigating reduction in hospital stay after laparoscopic colectomy			
Number of trials	Total number of patients	Significantly shorter length of stay than open	References
7	716	Yes	[35],[36],[37],[38],[41],[42],[43]

REFERENCES

1. Jacobs, M., Verdeja, J. C., and Goldstein, H. S. Minimally invasive colon resection (laparoscopic colectomy). *Surg Laparosc Endosc*, **1**:3 (1991), 144–50.
2. Bacha, E. A., Barber, W., and Ratchford, W. Port-site metastases of adenocarcinoma of the fallopian tube after laparoscopically assisted vaginal hysterectomy and salpingo-oophorectomy. *Surg Endosc*, **10**:11 (1996), 1102–3.

3. Cava, A., *et al.* Subcutaneous metastasis following laparoscopy in gastric adenocarcinoma. *Eur J Surg Oncol*, **16**:1 (1990), 63–7.

4. Dobronte, Z., Wittmann, T., and Karacsony, G. Rapid development of malignant metastases in the abdominal wall after laparoscopy. *Endoscopy*, **10**:2 (1978), 127–30.

5. Elbahnasy, A. M., *et al.* Laparoscopic staging of bladder tumor: concerns about port site metastases. *J Endourol*, **12**:1 (1998), 55–9.

6. Freeman, R. K. and Wait, M. A. Port site metastasis after laparoscopic staging of esophageal carcinoma. *Ann Thorac Surg*, **71**:3 (2001), 1032–4.

7. Kadar, N. Port-site recurrences following laparoscopic operations for gynaecological malignancies. *Br J Obstet Gynaecol*, **104**:11 (1997), 1308–13.

8. Morice, P., *et al.* Port-site metastasis after laparoscopic surgery for gynecologic cancer: a report of six cases. *J Reprod Med*, **45**:10 (2000), 837–40.

9. Muntz, H. G., *et al.* Port-site recurrence after laparoscopic surgery for endometrial carcinoma. *Obstet Gynecol*, **93**:5 Pt 2 (1999), 807–9.

10. Naumann, R. W. and Spencer, S. An umbilical metastasis after laparoscopy for squamous cell carcinoma of the cervix. *Gynecol Oncol*, **64**:3 (1997), 507–9.

11. Nduka, C. C., *et al.* Abdominal wall metastases following laparoscopy. *Br J Surg*, **81**:5 (1994), 648–52.

12. Russi, E. G., *et al.* Unusual relapse of hepatocellular carcinoma. *Cancer*, **70**:6 (1992), 1483–7.

13. Siriwardena, A. and Samarji, W. N. Cutaneous tumour seeding from a previously undiagnosed pancreatic carcinoma after laparoscopic cholecystectomy. *Ann R Coll Surg Engl*, **75**:3 (1993), 199–200.

14. Wang, P. H., *et al.* Risk factors contributing to early occurrence of port site metastases of laparoscopic surgery for malignancy. *Gynecol Oncol*, **72**:1 (1999), 38–44.

15. Wexner, S. D. and Cohen, S. M. Port site metastases after laparoscopic colorectal surgery for cure of malignancy. *Br J Surg*, **82**:3 (1995), 295–8.

16. Carter, J. J. and Whelan, R. L. The immunologic consequences of laparoscopy in oncology. *Surg Oncol Clin N Am*, **10**:3 (2001), 655–77.

17. Whelan, R. L., *et al.* Postoperative cell mediated immune response is better preserved after laparoscopic vs open colorectal resection in humans. *Surg Endosc*, **17**:6 (2003), 972–8.

18. Braga, M., *et al.* Laparoscopic vs. open colectomy in cancer patients: long-term complications, quality of life, and survival. *Dis Colon Rectum*, **48**:12 (2005), 2217–23.

19. Hazebroek, E. J. COLOR: a randomized clinical trial comparing laparoscopic and open resection for colon cancer. *Surg Endosc*, **16**:6 (2002), 949–53.

20. Chang, Y. J., *et al.* Hand-assisted laparoscopic sigmoid colectomy: helping hand or hindrance? *Surg Endosc*, **19**:5 (2005), 656–61.

21. HALSStudyGroup. Hand assisted laparoscopic surgery vs standard laparoscopic surgery for colorectal disease: a prospective randomised trial. *Surg Endosc*, **14**:10 (2000), 898–901.

22. Bemelman, W. A., *et al.* Laparoscopic-assisted colectomy with the dexterity pneumo sleeve. *Dis Colon Rectum*, **39**:suppl. 10 (1996), S59–61.

23. Darzi, A. Hand-assisted laparoscopic colorectal surgery. *Surg Endosc*, **14**:11 (2000), 999–1004.

24. Ichihara, T., *et al*. Laparoscopic lower anterior resection is equivalent to laparotomy for lower rectal cancer at the distal line of resection. *Am J Surg*, **179**:2 (2000), 97–8.

25. Miura, Y., *et al*. Gasless hand-assisted laparoscopic surgery for colorectal cancer: an option for poor cardiopulmonary reserve. *Dis Colon Rectum*, **44**:6 (2001), 896–8.

26. Nakajima, K., *et al*. Hand-assisted laparoscopic colorectal surgery using GelPort. *Surg Endosc*, **18**:1 (2004), 102–5.

27. Pietrabissa, A., *et al*. Hand-assisted laparoscopic low anterior resection: initial experience with a new procedure. *Surg Endosc*, **16**:3 (2002), 431–5.

28. Darzi, A., *et al*. Laparoscopic abdominoperineal excision of the rectum. *Surg Endosc*, **9**:4 (1995), 414–17.

29. Fowler, D. L. and White, S. A. Laparoscopy-assisted sigmoid resection. *Surg Laparosc Endosc*, **1**:3 (1991), 183–8.

30. Peters, W. R. and Bartels, T. L. Minimally invasive colectomy: are the potential benefits realized? *Dis Colon Rectum*, **36**:8 (1993), 751–6.

31. Phillips, E. H., *et al*. Laparoscopic colectomy. *Ann Surg*, **216**:6 (1992), 703–7.

32. Schlinkert, R. T. Laparoscopic-assisted right hemicolectomy. *Dis Colon Rectum*, **34**:11 (1991), 1030–1.

33. Scoggin, S. D., *et al*. Laparoscopic-assisted bowel surgery. *Dis Colon Rectum*, **36**:8 (1993), 747–50.

34. Delgado, S., *et al*. Could age be an indication for laparoscopic colectomy in colorectal cancer? *Surg Endosc*, **14**:1 (2000), 22–6.

35. Schwenk, W., Bohm, B., and Muller, J. M. Postoperative pain and fatigue after laparoscopic or conventional colorectal resections. A prospective randomized trial. *Surg Endosc*, **12**:9 (1998), 1131–6.

36. Curet, M. J., *et al*. Laparoscopically assisted colon resection for colon carcinoma: perioperative results and long-term outcome. *Surg Endosc*, **14**:11 (2000), 1062–6.

37. Hasegawa, H., *et al*. Randomized controlled trial of laparoscopic versus open colectomy for advanced colorectal cancer. *Surg Endosc*, **17**:4 (2003), 636–40.

38. Lacy, A. M., *et al*. Laparoscopy-assisted colectomy versus open colectomy for treatment of non-metastatic colon cancer: a randomised trial. *Lancet*, **359**:9325 (2002), 2224–9.

39. Milsom, J. W., *et al*. A prospective, randomized trial comparing laparoscopic versus conventional techniques in colorectal cancer surgery: a preliminary report. *J Am Coll Surg*, **187**:1 (1998), 46–54, discussion 54–5.

40. Vignali, A., *et al*. Laparoscopic vs. open colectomies in octogenarians: a case-matched control study. *Dis Colon Rectum*, **48**:11 (2005), 2070–5.

41. Weeks, J. C., *et al*. Short-term quality-of-life outcomes following laparoscopic-assisted colectomy vs open colectomy for colon cancer: a randomized trial. *JAMA*, **287**:3 (2002), 321–8.

42. Nelson, H. S., Fleshman, J. *et al*. Clinical outcomes of surgical therapy study group of the laparoscopic colectomy trial: a comparison of laparoscopically assisted and open colectomy for colon cancer. *N Engl J Med*, **350** (2004), 2050–9.

43. Stage, J. G., *et al*. Prospective randomized study of laparoscopic versus open colonic resection for adenocarcinoma. *Br J Surg*, **84**:3 (1997), 391–6.

44. Anderson, C. A., *et al*. Results of laparoscopically assisted colon resection for carcinoma. *Surg Endosc*, **16**:4 (2002), 607–10.

45. Schiedeck, T. H., *et al*. Laparoscopic surgery for the cure of colorectal cancer: results of a German five-center study. *Dis Colon Rectum*, **43**:1 (2000), 1–8.

46. Tsang, W. W., Chung, C. C., and Li, M. K. Prospective evaluation of laparoscopic total mesorectal excision with colonic J-pouch reconstruction for mid and low rectal cancers. *Br J Surg*, **90**:7 (2003), 867–71.

47. Zhou, Z. G., *et al*. Laparoscopic total mesorectal excision of low rectal cancer with preservation of anal sphincter: a report of 82 cases. *World J Gastroenterol*, **9**:7 (2003), 1477–81.

48. Kehlet, H. and Dahl, J. B. Anaesthesia, surgery, and challenges in postoperative recovery. *Lancet*, **362**:9399 (2003), 1921–8.

49. Kehlet, H. and Wilmore, D. W. Multimodal strategies to improve surgical outcome. *Am J Surg*, **183**:6 (2002), 630–41.

50. Bardram, L., Funch-Jensen, P., and Kehlet, H. Rapid rehabilitation in elderly patients after laparoscopic colonic resection. *Br J Surg*, **87**:11 (2000), 1540–5.

51. Senagore, A. J., *et al*. Results of a standardized technique and postoperative care plan for laparoscopic sigmoid colectomy: a 30-month experience. *Dis Colon Rectum*, **46**:4 (2003), 503–9.

52. Basse, L., *et al*. A clinical pathway to accelerate recovery after colonic resection. *Ann Surg*, **232**:1 (2000), 51–7.

53. Basse, L., *et al*. Functional recovery after open versus laparoscopic colonic resection: a randomized, blinded study. *Ann Surg*, **241**:3 (2005), 416–23.

54. Basse, L., *et al*. Accelerated postoperative recovery programme after colonic resection improves physical performance, pulmonary function and body composition. *Br J Surg*, **89**:4 (2002), 446–53.

55. King, P. M., *et al*. Randomized clinical trial comparing laparoscopic and open surgery for colorectal cancer within an enhanced recovery programme. *Br J Surg*, **93**:3 (2006), 300–8.

56. Decanini, C., *et al*. Laparoscopic oncologic abdominoperineal resection. *Dis Colon Rectum*, **37**:6 (1994), 552–8.

57. Franklin, M. E., Jr., *et al*. Prospective comparison of open vs. laparoscopic colon surgery for carcinoma. Five-year results. *Dis Colon Rectum*, **39**:suppl. 10 (1996), S35–46.

58. Lord, S. A., *et al*. Laparoscopic resections for colorectal carcinoma. A three-year experience. *Dis Colon Rectum*, **39**:2 (1996), 148–54.

59. Moore, J. W., *et al*. Lymphovascular clearance in laparoscopically assisted right hemicolectomy is similar to open surgery. *Aust N Z J Surg*, **66**:9 (1996), 605–7.

60. Abcarian, H. Operative treatment of colorectal cancer. *Cancer*, **70**:suppl. 5 (1992), 1350–4.

61. Corder, A. P., *et al*. Flush aortic tie versus selective preservation of the ascending left colic artery in low anterior resection for rectal carcinoma. *Br J Surg*, **79**:7 (1992), 680–2.

62. Bonjer, H. J., *et al*. [Abdominal wall metastasis following surgical removal of colorectal carcinomas]. *Ned Tijdschr Geneeskd*, **141**:39 (1997), 1868–70.

63. Lacy, A. M., *et al*. Port site metastases and recurrence after laparoscopic colectomy. A randomized trial. *Surg Endosc*, **12**:8 (1998), 1039–42.

64. Wittich, P., *et al*. [The 'Colon cancer laparoscopic or open resection' (COLOR) trial]. *Ned Tijdschr Geneeskd*, **141**:39 (1997), 1870–1.

65. O'Connell, M. Phase III randomised study of laparoscopic assisted colectomy versus open colectomy for colon cancer. Cancernet. Available at: http://cancernet.nci.nih.gov/. Accessed December 2004.

66. Guillou, P. J., *et al*. Short-term endpoints of conventional versus laparoscopic-assisted surgery in patients with colorectal cancer (MRC CLASICC trial): multicentre, randomised controlled trial. *Lancet*, **365**:9472 (2005), 1718–26.

67. Larach, S. W. and Gallagher, J. T. Complications of laparoscopic surgery for rectal cancer: avoidance and management. *Semin Surg Oncol*, **18**:3 (2000), 265–8.

68. Schrenk, P., *et al*. Mechanism, management, and prevention of laparoscopic bowel injuries. *Gastrointest Endosc*, **43**:6 (1996), 572–4.

69. Bateman, B. G., Kolp, L. A., and Hoeger, K. Complications of laparoscopy – operative and diagnostic. *Fertil Steril*, **66**:1 (1996), 30–5.

70. Jansen, F. W., *et al*. Complications of laparoscopy: an inquiry about closed- versus open-entry technique. *Am J Obstet Gynecol*, **190**:3 (2004), 634–8.

71. Schafer, M., Lauper, M., and Krahenbuhl, L. Trocar and Veress needle injuries during laparoscopy. *Surg Endosc*, **15**:3 (2001), 275–80.

72. Schafer, M. and Krahenbuhl, L. Effect of laparoscopy on intra-abdominal blood flow. *Surgery*, **129**:4 (2001), 385–9.

73. Chapron, C., *et al*. Surgical complications of diagnostic and operative gynaecological laparoscopy: a series of 29,966 cases. *Hum Reprod*, **13**:4 (1998), 867–72.

74. Kaali, S. G., Barad, D. H., and Merkatz, I. R. Avoiding trocar injuries – is there a fail-safe method? *Fertil Steril*, **66**:6 (1996), 1045–6.

75. Lewis, J. E. A simple technique for anticipating and managing secondary puncture site hemorrhage during laparoscopic surgery. A report of two cases. *J Reprod Med*, **40**:10 (1995), 729–30.

76. Nordestgaard, A. G., *et al*. Major vascular injuries during laparoscopic procedures. *Am J Surg*, **169**:5 (1995), 543–5.

77. Soderstrom, R. M. Injuries to major blood vessels during endoscopy. *J Am Assoc Gynecol Laparosc*, **4**:3 (1997), 395–8.

78. Heald, R. J. and Ryall, R. D. Recurrence and survival after total mesorectal excision for rectal cancer. *Lancet*, **1**:8496 (1986), 1479–82.

79. Hartley, J. E., *et al*. Patterns of recurrence and survival after laparoscopic and conventional resections for colorectal carcinoma. *Ann Surg*, **232**:2 (2000), 181–6.

80. Pearlstone, D. B., *et al*. Laparoscopy in 533 patients with abdominal malignancy. *Surgery*, **125**:1 (1999), 67–72.

81. Psaila, J., *et al*. Outcome following laparoscopic resection for colorectal cancer. *Br J Surg*, **85**:5 (1998), 662–4.

6

Chemotherapy

Yu Jo Chua and David Cunningham

Introduction

In the past decade, the systemic treatment options for advanced colorectal cancer have expanded from the use of single agent 5-fluorouracil (5FU) chemotherapy to three active cytotoxic agents (5FU and other fluoropyrimidine analogs, oxaliplatin, and irinotecan), as well as the novel targeted therapies, bevacizumab and cetuximab. With the different combination and treatment sequencing options available, patients with this disease are achieving median survivals in excess of 20 months in clinical trials [1,2,3,4,5]. The benefits observed from the use of combination treatment in metastatic disease have stimulated clinical trials in the adjuvant and neoadjuvant settings. Already, oxaliplatin in combination with 5FU has been shown to be beneficial in the adjuvant treatment of patients with stage II and III resected colon cancer [6,7]. In each setting, the radiologist has a key role to play in the selection of patients for different treatment strategies, monitoring the progress of patients on treatment, and surveillance of patients for relapse or recurrence after initial successful treatment.

Chemotherapy for advanced inoperable colorectal cancer

The systemic treatment of patients with colorectal cancer is regarded as palliative when their disease is found to be metastatic, or to be locally advanced and inoperable (Figure 6.1). In this setting, the aim of treatment is to achieve control of disease in order to prolong survival, with a particular emphasis on treating or preventing cancer-related symptoms and on maintaining quality of life. Despite advances in systemic therapy, treatment is not on its own likely to cure patients, although, as will be discussed later on, there is increasing interest in neoadjuvant treatment in which it is hoped that a subset of patients may be downstaged and rendered operable.

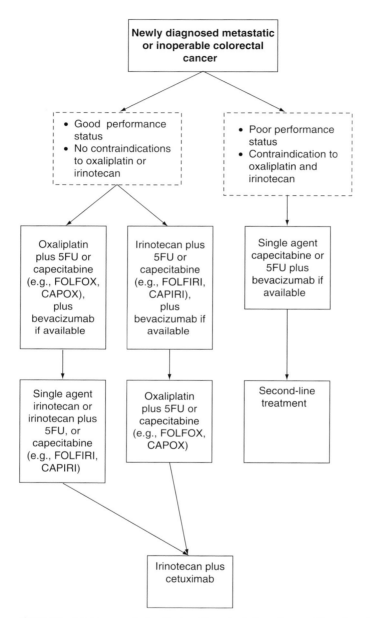

Figure 6.1   Management of patients with metastatic or inoperable colorectal cancer. The use of other chemotherapy agents such as mitomycin-C and raltitrexed has not been shown, but may be considered in certain clinical circumstances. Whenever possible, patients should be offered entry into a suitable clinical trial at any stage of treatment.

For several decades, the antimetabolite 5FU was the only effective treatment for advanced colorectal cancer [8,9,10,11,12]. Whilst many efforts were made to improve the outcomes of patients by modifying doses, schedules, and combining 5FU with modulators (such as leucovorin), median survivals beyond 12 months were rarely achieved. Since then, the third-generation platinum compound oxaliplatin and the semisynthetic campothecin irinotecan have been shown to be more efficacious when used in combination with 5FU than 5FU alone, and they have significantly improved the benefits of treatment when used in both the first- and second-line settings [3,13,14,15,16,17,18]. The oxaliplatin-based FOLFOX and the irinotecan-based FOLFIRI regimens were found to have similar efficacy when compared directly by Tournigand *et al.* [3], so that in clinical practice combinations based on either agent with a fluoropyrimidine such as 5FU or capecitabine are considered as acceptable treatments in the first-line setting. In the same study, patients were protocolized to receive the other chemotherapy combination on progression of disease, with both arms achieving some of the best results seen in chemotherapy trials in this disease so far, with the median survivals of both arms exceeding 20 months [3]. Irinotecan does however have single agent activity and has also been shown to be beneficial as second-line monotherapy [17]. A more important issue than the order in which these agents are used is that patients should receive all three active agents during the course of their disease. A meta-analysis by Grothey *et al.* has confirmed that these were the patients who achieved the longest median survivals in clinical trials [1,2].

Although combination chemotherapy is preferred as first-line treatment, it may not be appropriate for all patients, as it is potentially associated with an increased likelihood of toxicity in some patients. It would be reasonable to treat these patients with fluoropyrimidine monotherapy, either with 5FU and leucovorin or with capecitabine. The latter is an oral prodrug of 5FU which has similar efficacy to 5FU with the advantage of ease of administration [19].

More recently, the forefront of development in the treatment of colorectal cancer has shifted toward the use of the novel targeted agents, which are either monoclonal antibodies or small molecule tyrosine kinase inhibitors which antagonize various signaling pathways which promote the growth and development of cancer. In colorectal cancer, the agents which have been licensed for use are the monoclonal antibodies, bevacizumab, and cetuximab. Bevacizumab targets vascular endothelial growth factor (VEGF) and has been shown, in a randomized trial in the first-line setting, to significantly improve overall and progression-free survival, and response rate compared to chemotherapy alone [5]. Although initially evaluated with the irinotecan-based IFL regimen, there is also evidence that similar efficacy is seen with oxaliplatin, both in the first- and second-line settings [20,21]. Cetuximab blocks the epidermal growth factor receptor (EGFR), which is over-expressed in over 80% of colorectal cancers [22,23]. In patients with irinotecan refractory disease who were mostly heavily pretreated, cetuximab appears to reverse chemo-resistance when given together with irinotecan, resulting in an overall response rate of 22.9% [4]. More interestingly, the results of a recent phase II study reported an impressive response rate of 72% when cetuximab was added to FOLFOX4 in the first-line setting [24]. Whilst patients in clinical trials of cetuximab have been selected on the basis of the demonstration of EGFR positivity by immunohistochemistry, subsequent reports have shown that apparently EGFR negative patients also respond to treatment [25]. Therefore, EGFR status by immunohistochemistry should not be used to select patients for treatment. In most cases, both agents should be used in addition to chemotherapy.

A different profile of treatment-related toxicity has been observed with these agents compared to cytotoxic chemotherapy. In general, this has allowed these agents to be added to established chemotherapy regimens with only minimal or modest increases in toxicity. However, clinicians should be aware of these unique side effects, as they are managed differently to those of cytotoxic chemotherapy, and whilst in most part these agents are very well tolerated, they can sometimes have potentially life-threatening consequences. For example, well-known but uncommon adverse effects of bevacizumab are bowel perforation and an increased risk of arterial thromboembolism [26]. Other potential toxicities include impaired wound healing, bleeding, hypertension, and proteinuria. However, the outcomes of patients who have either commenced treatment after surgery or have had to have emergency surgery during treatment in the randomized trials in advanced disease suggest that an interval of 8 weeks between the last administration of bevacizumab and surgery and a minimum interval of 4 weeks from surgery to the commencement of postoperative bevacizumab should minimize the risk of perioperative complications related to the agent [27]. Cetuximab, in common with other inhibitors of the EGFR pathway, frequently causes a characteristic skin rash [4]. More recently recognized is an association between the agent and hypomagnesemia and lethargy [28].

- Either oxaliplatin or irinotecan in combination with 5FU or capecitabine are standard first-line treatment options for patients with advanced colorectal cancer. If available, bevacizumab should also be offered to these patients with combination chemotherapy.

- For patients who are unable to receive these standard chemotherapy combinations, suitable alternatives include a single agent fluoropyrimidine such as capecitabine or 5FU.
- Patients who are irinotecan refractory may benefit from the addition of cetuximab to irinotecan.

Adjuvant chemotherapy for resected early stage colorectal cancer

Chemotherapy is administered to patients with TNM stage III (node positive) disease, and some patients with stage II (node negative) disease, after surgery in order to reduce their risk of disease recurrence (Figure 6.2). The benefits of adjuvant chemotherapy with 5FU and Levimasole (as a modulator of 5FU) were initially demonstrated by Moertel *et al.* [29] in stage III patients, followed by the results of a study in stage II and III patients which showed that 5FU with Leucovorin improved disease-free and overall survival advantage compared to the MOF regimen (lomustine, vincristine, and 5FU) [30]. Whereas the use of adjuvant chemotherapy was recommended by the US National Institute of Health 1990 Consensus Conference in patients with stage III disease on the basis of such evidence from clinical trials [31], the benefit in stage II patients has been more difficult to prove and has been the subject of several meta-analysis [32,33,34]. However, in a non-randomized subgroup comparison in the UK QUASAR study, a small benefit in favor of chemotherapy was observed in these patients [35]. The American Society of Clinical Oncology guidelines on adjuvant treatment for patients with stage II colon cancer concluded that although direct evidence did not support routine in this group of patients, benefit for these patients could still be inferred from that observed in stage III patients [36]. Therefore, some patients with stage II disease should still be considered for adjuvant treatment, in particular those with high-risk disease, defined in the guidelines as the presence of adverse prognostic factors such as poorly differentiated or T4-stage histology, inadequate lymph node harvesting at surgery (less than 13 negative lymph nodes), extra-mural venous invasion or presentation with perforation. Postoperative adjuvant treatment is also routinely used in patients with resected rectal cancer. A benefit for these patients was also observed in the QUASAR study [35].

More recently, two randomized trials (MOSAIC and US NSABP C-07) have shown that the addition of oxaliplatin to 5FU adjuvant chemotherapy improves

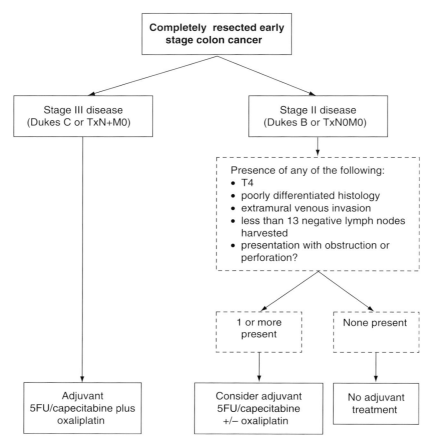

Figure 6.2 Postoperative adjuvant treatment for patients with resected early stage colon cancer.

3-year disease-free survival (the primary end point of both these studies) in patients with resected stage II and III colon cancer [6,7]. The license for oxaliplatin has been extended to adjuvant treatment for stage III disease on the basis of these results. On the other hand, two randomized trials of irinotecan-based combination chemotherapy failed to demonstrate a statistically significant improvement in disease-free survival [37,38]. Whether a survival difference will be observed with longer follow-up is not yet known.

- Patients with resected stage III colon cancer should be offered postoperative oxaliplatin-based combination adjuvant chemotherapy.
- The use of adjuvant treatment in patients with stage II disease should be considered on a case-by-case basis; it should be considered in patients with high-risk features.

Neoadjuvant or preoperative treatment

Two settings in colorectal cancer in which neoadjuvant treatment is used are in the management of locally advanced rectal cancer and as downstaging treatment for patients with initially unresectable isolated liver metastases. Both are highly dependent on an effective multidisciplinary management approach for success, and radiology plays a particularly central role in selecting patients for different treatment strategies, in particular with magnetic resonance imaging techniques. A detailed discussion of selection criteria is beyond the scope of this chapter, as they have been differently defined in various studies.

In locally advanced rectal cancer, preoperative treatment based on radiotherapy is standard treatment, whether it is so-called "short-course treatment" (25 Gy given in 5 Gy fractions over 5 days followed soon after by surgery) [39,40,41] or "hyperfractionated chemoradiotherapy" (45–56 Gy in 1.8 Gy fractions of radiotherapy over 5–6 weeks with a concurrent fluoropyrimidine) [42,43,44,45]. These have generally resulted in reductions in local recurrence rates without improving overall survival, hence the interest in developing treatment strategies with combination systemic chemotherapy given with radiotherapy. Another experimental approach has been to use neoadjuvant chemotherapy prior to chemoradiotherapy [46]. Whilst definitions vary, patients may be considered to have locally advanced disease on the basis of factors such as T3 or greater stage tumors, involvement of regional lymph nodes (N+ disease) or extramural venous invasion, low tumors (less than 6 cm from the anal verge), or threatened or involved circumferential resection margins. The management of these patients is summarized in Figure 6.3.

The use of downstaging chemotherapy is appealing in patients with initially unresectable liver metastases as these patients form a significant proportion of patients who would otherwise be treated with palliative intent. The evidence supporting the feasibility and benefits of treatment is derived from several large case series and a number of small non-randomized trials [47,48,49,50,51]. Up to 50% of these patients have become resectable with curative intent after treatment with either oxaliplatin- or irinotecan-based combination chemotherapy, with an overall survival rate of up to 40% at 5 years reported in completely resected patients, exceeding outcomes achieved in most patients with chemotherapy alone. Criteria for unresectability of liver metastases tend to be based on the presence of adverse prognostic features (such as synchronous presentation of metastases with the primary disease, size of largest metastasis, number of metastases, bilobar involvement, or extra-hepatic metastases), technical factors (such as metastasis closely adjacent to

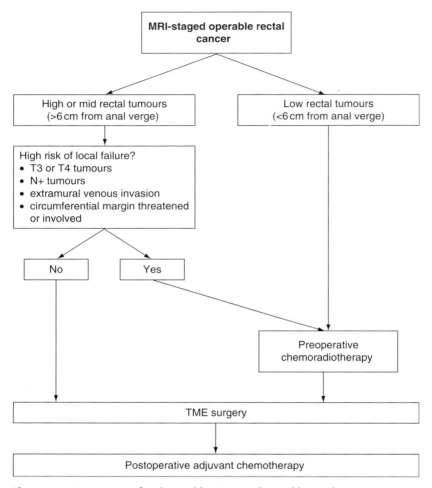

Figure 6.3   Management of patients with MRI-staged operable rectal cancer.

or involving major vascular structures), and involvement of more than 70% of liver parenchyma (at least 30% of residual normal functioning liver parenchyma is required to avoid postoperative liver failure). The benefit of neoadjuvant chemotherapy in patients with initially resectable metastases is less well known, and is the subject of a randomized trial for which efficacy results are expected in 2006 [52].

● The use of preoperative treatment is standard in patients with locally advanced rectal cancer. This includes the use of chemoradiotherapy. Pretreatment MRI staging is important to prevent the over-treatment of patients with better prognosis disease.

● Whilst current evidence supports the use of downstaging combination chemotherapy in patients with initially unresectable isolated liver metastases from colorectal cancer, these patients should be treated within clinical trials where possible as the role and benefits of this treatment strategy need to be better defined.

Conclusions

Systemic chemotherapy is the main therapeutic option for patients with advanced colorectal cancer, and for many patients with resectable disease, with recent advances seen with the use of combination cytotoxics chemotherapy and the additional use of the novel targeted agents. However, patients should be treated within a multidisciplinary setting in which the most appropriate treatment strategy for a given patient's situation can be decided, making optimal use of the expanded management options already available.

Where possible, suitably fit patients with previously untreated advanced colorectal cancer should be treated with combination chemotherapy with either oxaliplatin or irinotecan. Patients who progress after first-line treatment should receive further treatment with non-cross resistant combination chemotherapy, with a view to ensuring exposure to the three active cytotoxics agents. In many countries, the targeted agents are also in routine use, with bevacizumab in the first-line setting, and cetuximab in irinotecan refractory disease, although ongoing clinical trials may also show these agents to be useful in other disease settings. Patients who are unable to receive combination chemotherapy with oxaliplatin or irinotecan can still be considered for treatment with better tolerated combinations, or with monotherapy with a fluoropyrimidine.

Adjuvant chemotherapy is standard for all patients with stage III resected colon cancer. Patients without contraindications should be offered treatment with oxaliplatin-based combination chemotherapy. In patients with stage II disease, however, the issues of whether adjuvant treatment is appropriate, and if so, whether monotherapy or combination, should be considered on a case-by-case basis depending on the presence of adverse prognostic factors, with a discussion with the patient about the likely benefits and risks of treatment in their case.

REFERENCES

1. Grothey, A., Sargent, D., Goldberg, R. M., *et al*. Survival of patients with advanced colorectal cancer improves with the availability of fluorouracil-leucovorin, irinotecan, and oxaliplatin in the course of treatment. *J Clin Oncol*, **22** (2004), 1209–14.

2. Grothey, A. and Sargent, D. Overall survival of patients with advanced colorectal cancer (CRC) correlates with availability of 5-fluorouracil, irinotecan and oxaliplatin regardless of whether doublet or single agent therapy is used first-line. *Program and Proceedings of the 2006 Gastrointestinal Cancers Symposium* (San Francisco, California, 2006), abstract, 282.

3. Tournigand, C., Andre, T., Achille, E., *et al.* FOLFIRI followed by FOLFOX6 or the reverse sequence in advanced colorectal cancer: a randomized GERCOR study. *J Clin Oncol*, **22** (2004), 229–37.

4. Cunningham, D., Humblet, Y., Siena, S., *et al.* Cetuximab monotherapy and cetuximab plus irinotecan in irinotecan-refractory metastatic colorectal cancer. *N Engl J Med*, **351** (2004), 337–45.

5. Hurwitz, H., Fehrenbacher, L., Novotny, W., *et al.* Bevacizumab plus irinotecan, fluorouracil, and leucovorin for metastatic colorectal cancer. *N Engl J Med*, **350** (2004), 2335–42.

6. Andre, T., Boni, C., Mounedji-Boudiaf, L., *et al.* Oxaliplatin, fluorouracil, and leucovorin as adjuvant treatment for colon cancer. *N Engl J Med*, **350** (2004), 2343–51.

7. Wolmark, N., Wieand, H. S., Kuebler, J. P., *et al.* A phase III trial comparing FULV to FULV + oxaliplatin in stage II or III carcinoma of the colon: results of NSABP Protocol C-07. *J Clin Oncol*, **23** (2005), abstr LBA3500.

8. Modulation of fluorouracil by leucovorin in patients with advanced colorectal cancer: evidence in terms of response rate. Advanced Colorectal Cancer Meta-Analysis Project. *J Clin Oncol*, **10** (1992), 896–903.

9. Meta-analysis of randomized trials testing the biochemical modulation of fluorouracil by methotrexate in metastatic colorectal cancer. Advanced Colorectal Cancer Meta-Analysis Project. *J Clin Oncol*, **12** (1994), 960–9.

10. Efficacy of intravenous continuous infusion of fluorouracil compared with bolus administration in advanced colorectal cancer. Meta-analysis Group in Cancer. *J Clin Oncol*, **16** (1998), 301–8.

11. Kohne, C. H., Wils, J., Lorenz, M., *et al.* Randomized phase III study of high-dose fluorouracil given as a weekly 24-hour infusion with or without leucovorin versus bolus fluorouracil plus leucovorin in advanced colorectal cancer: European Organization for Research and Treatment of Cancer Gastrointestinal Group Study 40952. *J Clin Oncol*, **21** (2003), 3721–8.

12. Piedbois, P. and Buyse, M. What can we learn from a meta-analysis of trials testing the modulation of 5-FU by leucovorin? Advanced Colorectal Meta-analysis Project. *Ann Oncol*, **4**:suppl. 2 (1993), 15–19.

13. de Gramont, A., Figer, A., Seymour, M., *et al.* Leucovorin and fluorouracil with or without oxaliplatin as first-line treatment in advanced colorectal cancer. *J Clin Oncol*, **18** (2000), 2938–47.

14. Douillard, J. Y., Cunningham, D., Roth, A. D., *et al.* Irinotecan combined with fluorouracil compared with fluorouracil alone as first-line treatment for metastatic colorectal cancer: a multicentre randomised trial. *Lancet*, **355** (2000), 1041–7.

15. Kohne, C. H., van Cutsem, E., Wils, J., *et al.* Phase III study of weekly high-dose infusional fluorouracil plus folinic acid with or without irinotecan in patients with metastatic colorectal

cancer: European Organisation for Research and Treatment of Cancer Gastrointestinal Group Study 40986. *J Clin Oncol*, **23** (2005), 4856–65.

16. Goldberg, R. M., Sargent, D. J., Morton, R. F., *et al.* A randomized controlled trial of fluorouracil plus leucovorin, irinotecan, and oxaliplatin combinations in patients with previously untreated metastatic colorectal cancer. *J Clin Oncol*, **22** (2004), 23–30.

17. Cunningham, D., Pyrhonen, S., James, R. D., *et al.* Randomised trial of irinotecan plus supportive care versus supportive care alone after fluorouracil failure for patients with metastatic colorectal cancer. *Lancet*, **352** (1998), 1413–18.

18. Saltz, L. B., Cox, J. V., Blanke, C., *et al.* Irinotecan plus fluorouracil and leucovorin for metastatic colorectal cancer. Irinotecan Study Group. *N Engl J Med*, **343** (2000), 905–14.

19. Van Cutsem, E., Twelves, C., Cassidy, J., *et al.* Oral capecitabine compared with intravenous fluorouracil plus leucovorin in patients with metastatic colorectal cancer: results of a large phase III study. *J Clin Oncol*, **19** (2001), 4097–106.

20. Giantonio, B. J., Catalano, P. J., Meropol, N. J., *et al.* High-dose bevacizumab improves survival when combined with FOLFOX4 in previously treated advanced colorectal cancer: results from the Eastern Cooperative Oncology Group (ECOG) study E3200. *J Clin Oncol*, **23**:suppl. 1 (2005), abstr 2.

21. Hochster, H. S., Welles, L., Hart, L., *et al.* Safety and efficacy of bevacizumab (Bev) when added to oxaliplatin/fluoropyrimidine (O/F) regimens as first-line treatment of metastatic colorectal cancer (mCRC): TREE 1 & 2 Studies. *J Clin Oncol*, **23**:suppl. 249 (2005), abstr 3515.

22. Yarden, Y. and Sliwkowski, M. X. Untangling the ErbB signalling network. *Nat Rev Mol Cell Biol*, **2** (2001), 127–37.

23. Spano, J. P., Lagorce, C., Atlan, D., *et al.* Impact of EGFR expression on colorectal cancer patient prognosis and survival. *Ann Oncol*, **16** (2005), 102–8.

24. Díaz Rubio, E., Tabernero, J., van Cutsem, E., *et al.* Cetuximab in combination with oxaliplatin/ 5-fluorouracil (5-FU)/folinic acid (FA) (FOLFOX-4) in the first-line treatment of patients with epidermal growth factor receptor (EGFR)-expressing metastatic colorectal cancer: an international phase II study. *J Clin Oncol*, **23** (2005), abstr 3535.

25. Chung, K. Y., Shia, J., Kemeny, N. E., *et al.* Cetuximab shows activity in colorectal cancer patients with tumors that do not express the epidermal growth factor receptor by immunohistochemistry. *J Clin Oncol*, **23** (2005), 1803–10.

26. Gordon, M. S., Cunningham, D. Managing patients treated with bevacizumab combination therapy. *Oncology*, **69**:suppl. 3 (2005), 25–33.

27. Scappaticci, F. A., Fehrenbacher, L., Cartwright, T., *et al.* Surgical wound healing complications in metastatic colorectal cancer patients treated with bevacizumab. *J Surg Oncol*, **91** (2005), 173–80.

28. Schrag, D., Chung, K. Y., Flombaum, C., *et al.* Cetuximab therapy and symptomatic hypomagnesemia. *J Natl Cancer Inst*, **97** (2005), 1221–4.

29. Moertel, C. G., Fleming, T. R., Macdonald, J. S., *et al.* Levamisole and fluorouracil for adjuvant therapy of resected colon carcinoma. *N Engl J Med*, **322** (1990), 352–8.

30. Wolmark, N., Rockette, H., Fisher, B., *et al.* The benefit of leucovorin-modulated fluorouracil as postoperative adjuvant therapy for primary colon cancer: results from National Surgical Adjuvant Breast and Bowel Project protocol C-03. *J Clin Oncol*, **11** (1993), 1879–87.

31. NIH consensus conference. Adjuvant therapy for patients with colon and rectal cancer. *Jama*, **264** (1990), 1444–50.

32. Efficacy of adjuvant fluorouracil and folinic acid in B2 colon cancer. International Multicentre Pooled Analysis of B2 Colon Cancer Trials (IMPACT B2) Investigators. *J Clin Oncol*, **17** (1999), 1356–63.

33. Figueredo, A., Charette, M. L., Maroun, J., *et al.* Adjuvant therapy for stage II colon cancer: a systematic review from the Cancer Care Ontario Program in evidence-based care's gastrointestinal cancer disease site group. *J Clin Oncol*, **22** (2004), 3395–407.

34. Mamounas, E., Wieand, S., Wolmark, N., *et al.* Comparative efficacy of adjuvant chemotherapy in patients with Dukes' B versus Dukes' C colon cancer: results from four National Surgical Adjuvant Breast and Bowel Project adjuvant studies (C-01, C-02, C-03, and C-04). *J Clin Oncol*, **17** (1999), 1349–55.

35. Gray, R. G., Barnwell, J., Hills, R., *et al.* QUASAR: a randomised study of adjuvant chemotherapy (CT) vs observation including 3238 colorectal cancer patients. *Proc Am Soc Clin Oncol*, **23**:246 (2004), abstr 3501.

36. Benson, A. B., 3rd, Schrag, D., Somerfield, M. R., *et al.* American Society of Clinical Oncology recommendations on adjuvant chemotherapy for stage II colon cancer. *J Clin Oncol*, **22** (2004), 3408–19.

37. Ychou, M., Raoul, J. L., Douillard, J. Y., *et al.* A phase III randomized trial of LV5FU2+CPT-11 vs. LV5FU2 alone in adjuvant high risk colon cancer (FNCLCC Accord02/FFCD9802). *J Clin Oncol*, **23**:suppl. 246 (2005), abstr 3502.

38. van Cutsem, E., Labianca, R., Hossfeld, D., *et al.* Randomized phase III trial conparing infused irintecan/5-fluorouracil (5-FU)/folinic acid (IF) versus 5-FU/DA (F) in stage III colon cancer patients (pts). *J Clin Oncol*, **23**:suppl. 3 (2005), abstr LBA8.

39. Kapiteijn, E., Marijnen, C. A., Nagtegaal, I. D., *et al.* Preoperative radiotherapy combined with total mesorectal excision for resectable rectal cancer. *N Engl J Med*, **345** (2001), 638–46.

40. Marijnen, C. A., Peeters, K., Putter, H., *et al.* Long term results, toxicity and quality of life in the TME trial. Program and Proceedings of the 2005 Gastrointestinal Cancers Sympossium, Hollywood, Florida (2005), abstr 166.

41. Swedish Rectal Cancer Trial: improved survival with preoperative radiotherapy in resectable rectal cancer. *N Engl J Med*, **336** (1997), 980–7.

42. Roh, M. S., Colangelo, L., Wieand, S., *et al.* Response to preoperative multimodality therapy predicts survival in patients with carcinoma of the rectum. *Proc Am Soc Clin Oncol*, **22**:suppl. 246 (2004), abstr 3505.

43. Sauer, R., Becker, H., Hohenberger, W., *et al.* Preoperative versus postoperative chemoradiotherapy for rectal cancer. *N Engl J Med*, **351** (2004), 1731–40.

44. Gerard, J., Bonnetain, F., Conroy, T., *et al.* Preoperative (preop) radiotherapy (RT) + 5 FU/ folinic acid (FA) in T3-4 rectal cancers : results of the FFCD 9203 randomized trial. *Proc Am Soc Clin Oncol,* **23**:suppl. 247 (2005), abstr 3504.

45. Bosset, J. F., Calais, G., Mineur, L., *et al.* Enhanced tumorocidal effect of chemotherapy with preoperative radiotherapy for rectal cancer: preliminary results – EORTC 22921. *J Clin Oncol,* **23** (2005), 5620–7.

46. Chau, I., Brown, G., Cunningham, D., *et al.* Neoadjuvant capecitabine and oxaliplatin followed by synchronous chemoradiation and total mesorectal excision in magnetic resonance imaging-defined poor-risk rectal cancer. *J Clin Oncol,* **24** (2006), 668–74.

47. Adam, R., Avisar, E., Ariche, A., *et al.* Five-year survival following hepatic resection after neoadjuvant therapy for nonresectable colorectal. *Ann Surg Oncol,* **8** (2001), 347–53.

48. Alberts, S. R., Horvath, W. L., Sternfeld, W. C., *et al.* Oxaliplatin, fluorouracil, and leucovorin for patients with unresectable liver-only metastases from colorectal cancer: a North Central Cancer Treatment Group phase II study. *J Clin Oncol,* **23** (2005), 9243–9.

49. Bismuth, H., Adam, R., Levi, F., *et al.* Resection of nonresectable liver metastases from colorectal cancer after neoadjuvant chemotherapy. *Ann Surg,* **224** (1996), 509–20, discussion 520–2.

50. Giacchetti, S., Itzhaki, M., Gruia, G., *et al.* Long-term survival of patients with unresectable colorectal cancer liver metastases following infusional chemotherapy with 5-fluorouracil, leucovorin, oxaliplatin and surgery. *Ann Oncol,* **10** (1999), 663–9.

51. Pozzo, C., Basso, M., Cassano, A., *et al.* Neoadjuvant treatment of unresectable liver disease with irinotecan and 5-fluorouracil plus folinic acid in colorectal cancer patients. *Ann Oncol,* **15** (2004), 933–9.

52. Nordlinger, B., Sorbye, H., Debois, M., *et al.* Feasibility and risks of pre-operative chemotherapy (CT) with Folfox 4 and surgery for resectable colorectal cancer liver metastases (LM). Interim results of the EORTC Intergroup randomized phase III study 40983. *J Clin Oncol,* **23** (2005), abstr 3528.

7

Radiotherapy in colorectal cancer

Brian D. P. O'Neill and Diana M. Tait

Patterns of failure

The patterns of failure of rectal cancer are crucial in the design of RT volumes. The best known pre-TME (total mesorectal excision) "map" of recurrences comes from Leonard Gunderson in the 1970s (Figure 7.1) [1]. This and other pre-TME series [2,3,4] imply that local mesorectal nodal and tumor bed recurrences outweigh the contribution of pelvic nodal disease. This pattern may have changed somewhat in the TME era, though this has not been reliably documented. Hocht *et al.* published recurrence data in 2002 from a series of 123 cases of recurrent rectal cancer [5] (Figure 7.2). Unfortunately, not all patients could be guaranteed to have had a TME, MRI was used in only a third, 17% had been treated with adjuvant RT.

The Dutch Colorectal Group has presented recurrence data after 5 years of follow-up. Like the Hocht data, this illustrates that lower tumors requiring an APE can recur high in the pelvis, though a new superior field border seemed possible in some patients (especially tumors 5–10 cm from the anal verge).

Technique

The volume covered by pelvic RT for rectal cancer includes the tumor bed with a margin, the mesentery, and perirectal, presacral, internal and common iliac lymph nodes. The anterior margin is increased to include external iliac nodes if the primary tumor invaded bladder, prostate, cervix, or vagina. The posterior margin includes the sacrum. Lateral margins include pelvic side-wall nodes. Superior margins are in the region of the L5/S1 interspace, and the inferior border depends

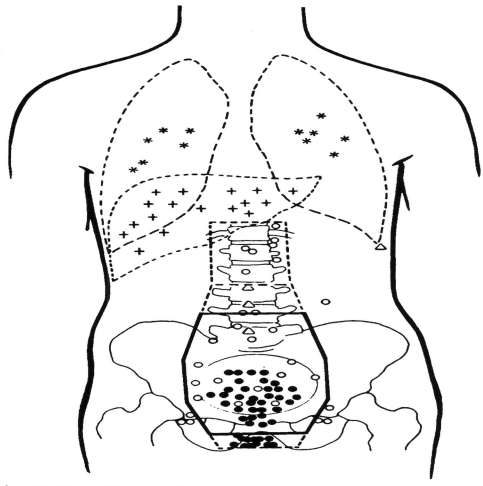

Figure 7.1 Patterns of failure of rectal cancer following initial operative procedure with superimposed radiation field. * = lung metastasis, + = liver metastasis, ● = local failure, ○ = lymph node involvement (courtesy of Leonard Gunderson [1]).

upon the level of tumor within the rectum. It is possible to spare the muscles of the anal sphincter for higher tumors.

The dose to this volume is usually 45 Gy in 25 fractions at 1.8 Gy per fraction over 5 weeks. Modern 3D computerized planning uses multiple fields and customized blocking to deliver high-dose radiation while reducing dose to normal tissues such as small bowel. A 3-field technique (1 posterior and 2 lateral fields) is typical, though a 4-field technique may also be used (Figure 7.3). A "boost" to

(A)

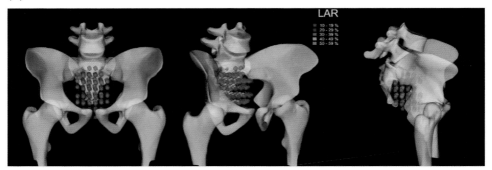

(B)

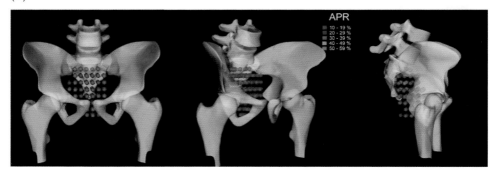

Figure 7.2   The representations shown are of sites of recurrence, with areas involved in < 10% of recurrences excluded, to illustrate a reasonable RT portal, after (A) LAR and (B) APE.

inoperable disease is delivered in some departments, to treat assessable primary tumor and nodal disease (via MRI, CT, and clinical examination) to a dose of 50.4 Gy, or 54 Gy if small bowel is excluded (Figure 7.4).

Pre- vs. postoperative radiotherapy

Postoperative RT [6,7] or CRT [8,9] was the standard of care for many years for stage II and III rectal cancer. Preoperative radiotherapy has a number of theoretical advantages over postoperative treatment. A less hypoxic tumor bed is presented, which improves the therapeutic ratio. The risk of tumor "spillage" during surgery may be reduced by preoperative sterilization of malignant cells. Small bowel settles deeper into the pelvis postoperatively, and becomes fixed by adhesions, increasing exposure, and likely toxicity. Neoadjuvant therapy offers the opportunity for

(A)

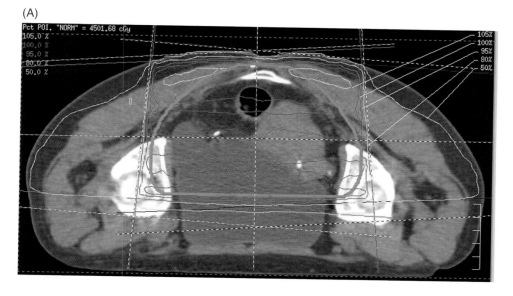

(B)

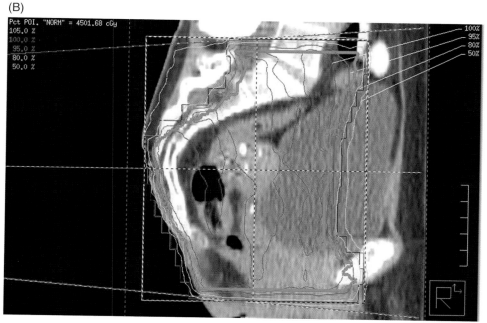

Figure 7.3 (A) Axial and (B) Sagittal phase I planning CT showing field arrangement and isodose distribution. The thickened line represents the Planning Target Volume phase I. In this example, note a higher superior border (standard is at the L5/S1 interspace) to cover a recto-sigmoid tumor with a 3-cm margin. Highlighted are 105%, 100%, 95%, 80%, and 50% isodoses.

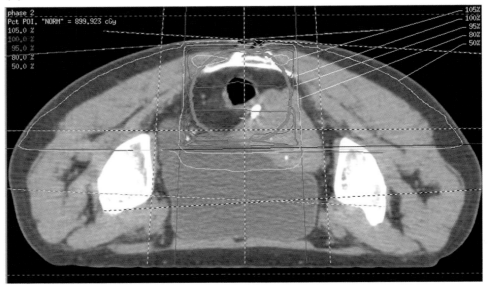

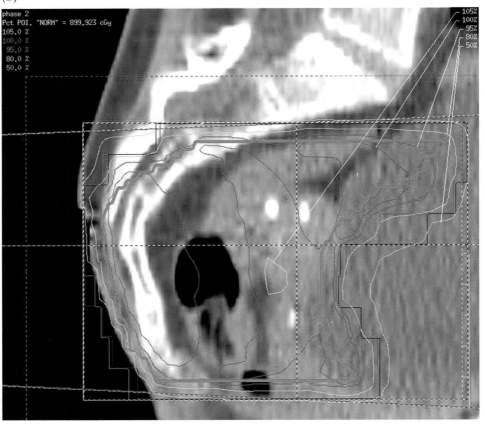

Figure 7.4 **(A) Axial and (B) Sagittal phase II planning CT showing (typical anterior and wedged laterals) field arrangement and isodose distribution. The thickened line represents the Planning Target Volume phase II. Highlighted are 105%, 100%, 95%, 80% and 50% isodoses.**

"downstaging," and may facilitate sphincter preservation. Postoperative CRT may still be occasionally required for a close or positive margin, but all such patients should ideally receive preoperative therapy.

Two prospective randomized trials, NSABP R-03 [10] and INT 1047, compared pre- and postoperative CRT for patients with locally advanced rectal tumors. Unfortunately, both were closed owing to low accrual. The recently published German CAO/ARO/AIO-94 trial successfully randomized 823 patients with T3, T4, or node-positive rectal cancers within 16 cm of the anal verge to preoperative or postoperative therapy [11]. Preoperative treatment consisted of 50.4 Gy in 28 fractions with continuous infusion 5-Fluorouracil 1000 mg/m^2 daily for the first and fifth weeks of radiotherapy. The postoperative arm received the same CRT, though an additional 5.4-Gy boost was delivered to the tumor bed. Four 5-day cycles of bolus 5-Fluorouracil 500 mg/m^2 daily four weeks apart were administered adjuvantly either 1 month after surgery in the preoperative CRT arm, or 1 month following CRT in the postoperative CRT arm.

Five-year cumulative local relapse was 6% vs. 13% in favor of preoperative CRT ($p = 0.006$). Grade III and IV acute (27% vs. 40%, $p = 0.001$) and chronic (14% vs. 24%, $p = 0.01$) toxicities were more frequent in the postoperative arm. Overall survival was equivalent (76% vs. 74%, $p = 0.80$).

Short-course preoperative radiotherapy

"Short course" preoperative RT (SCPRT) is delivered on a neoadjuvant basis, 5 Gy daily over 5 days (Table 7.1). From a radiobiological standpoint, even allowing for its high dose per fraction, this represents a lower dose than a standard regimen (45–50.4 Gy at 1.8–2.0 Gy per fraction). SCPRT is appealing in that a reduction in the time required for delivery of RT may result in a superior outcome, combating the effects of accelerated cellular repopulation, a phenomenon displayed by malignant cells exposed to RT.

The Swedish rectal cancer trial is the only randomized study to demonstrate a survival advantage for the addition of radiotherapy to surgery [12]. From 1987 to 1990, 1147 eligible patients with resectable tumors below the sacral promontory were randomly assigned to RT (5 Gy daily over 5 days) followed by surgery within 7 days or surgery only. Five-year overall survival was 54% vs. 48% ($p = 0.004$). Local recurrence rate was 11% vs. 27% ($p = 0.001$), and this advantage was evident for all Duke's stages.

Table 7.1 Selected trials of neoadjuvant therapy and sphincter preservation

Trial	n	RT	Chemotherapy	Stage	Position	Sphincter saving procedure
Lyon 90–01	201	39 Gy (@ 1.3 Gy/ fraction) (Randomized to 2 week or 6–8 week interval from RT to Surgery)	No	T2-3	1–11 cm from anal verge	68% short interval, 76% long interval ($p = 0.27$)
German Rectal Cancer Study Group	800	Randomized 50.4 Gy pre-op vs. 50.4 Gy post-op + 5.4 Gy boost	5-FU continuous infusion 1000 mg/ (m^2 day) first and fifth week	T3-4 N0-1	Within 16 cm of anal verge	194 assigned to APE pre-randomization, 39% vs. 19% ($p = 0.004$)
MSK	27	50.4 Gy	No (some had adjuvant)	T2N0	All assigned APE	78%
K. Bujko et al.	316	Randomized to 5 × 5 Gy vs. 50.4 Gy	No for 5 × 5 Gy arm; 5-FU 325 mg/(m^2 day) rapid infusion first and fifth week	T3-4	Palpable on DRE	61% vs. 58% ($p = 0.57$)
Lyon R96–02	90	Randomized 39 Gy vs. 39 Gy + 85 Gy Boost CXT 50 kV ± 25 Gy Brachytherapy boost	No	T2 T3 NX	6 cm from anal verge Not involving >Two-thirds circumference	76% vs. 44% ($p = 0.004$)

Some years later, the Dutch Colorectal Cancer Group investigated the combination of total mesorectal excision (TME) and short-course preoperative RT [13]. Again all non-metastatic resectable stages were eligible (28% stage I). 1805 patients with tumors within 15 cm of the anal verge were randomized to neoadjuvant $5\,Gy \times 5$ and TME vs. TME alone. Surgery was performed within 10 days following completion of RT. Overall survival at 2 years was 82.0% vs. 81.8%. Local recurrence rate at 2 years was 2.4% vs. 8.2% ($p < 0.001$). Stages II and III enjoyed a definite local control advantage, though unlike the Swedish trial, a trend was only observed for stage I disease ($p = 0.15$).

The Dutch Colorectal Group have shown neither short-course preoperative RT (SCPRT, see below) nor postoperative long-course RT compensate for a positive circumferential resection margin (CRM), though there is a strong trend for a local control advantage for SCPRT with subsequent positive CRM (9.3% vs. 16.4%, $p = 0.08$) [14].

Concerns regarding the routine use of SCPRT are the omission of radiosensitizing chemotherapy [15], inclusion of all stages, and increased late toxicity. Despite downsizing (mean diameter 4.5 cm vs. 4 cm, $p < 0.001$), no significant downstaging effect is experienced, and thus SCPRT may not be utilized for sphincter-preserving strategies.

At the 2006 annual meeting of the American Society of Clinical Oncology, preliminary 3-year results of the Medical Research Council randomized trial CR-07 were presented [16]. Between 1998 and 2005, 1350 patients from 80 international centers (though predominantly in the UK) were enrolled. Operable non-metastatic rectal adenocarcinomas were randomized to non-selective SCPRT and surgery, or surgery followed by selective adjuvant CRT for CRM-positive patients only. Adjuvant chemotherapy was delivered as per local policy.

Local recurrence at 3 years is in favor of the SCPRT arm, 5% vs. 11% (Hazard ratio (HR) = 2.47, 95% Confidence Interval (CI) 1.61–3.70; $p < 0.0001$). Disease-free survival shows a 5% absolute difference from 75% to 80% at 3 years ($p = 0.03$), again in favor of the SCPRT arm. Overall survival was not significant (79% vs. 81%). These results look set to become more pronounced at 5 years, and it is possible that overall survival will become significant. A local recurrence advantage in the SCPRT arm was significant for all stages and levels of the rectum (in contrast with the Dutch study), and for CRM-negative disease (3% vs. 10%, HR 2.91, 95% CI 1.74–4.88). Patients with CRM-positive disease had an overall clear local recurrence disadvantage, but did not reach significance between the treatment arms, as a relatively small number ($n = 193$) had CRM-positive tumors (16% vs. 23%, HR 1.56, 95% CI 0.60–4.04).

Macroscopic evaluation of resection specimens, as described by Quirke, was applied to all specimens [17]. Of all specimens, 53% were considered high-quality TMEs. Overall, those patients that received high-quality TME showed a 1% vs. 6% local recurrence advantage in favor of SCPRT. Stage by stage breakdown of this group is awaited. This data will challenge clinicians to decide what level of local recurrence is considered "acceptable." For example, for all stage I disease, local recurrence of 3% at 3 years was reduced to 0% by SCPRT. While this was a significant result (HR 12.19, 95% CI 1.64–9.41), many clinicians would conclude that this level of recurrence risk would not merit the toxicity of SCPRT. Mature results are eagerly awaited.

There is only one randomized comparison between selective SCPRT (all previous SCPRT trials were non-selective) and selective standard "long-course" CRT [18]. Resectable palpable T3/4 tumors (n = 316) were randomly assigned to SCPRT or CRT at standard fractionation and dose with concomitant infusional 5-Fluorouracil 325 mg/m^2 daily for the first and fifth weeks of radiotherapy. The intervals between completion of RT and surgery were standard for each approach, 7 days for short course and 4–6 weeks for long course. No significant difference was found for either approach for patients with T3/4 rectal adenocarcinomas. Toxicity was similar for each approach.

Resectable locally advanced disease

It is now appreciated that the margin of excision and risk of a positive circumferential resection margin (CRM) can be accurately predicted by high spatial resolution preoperative MRI [19]. In some institutions, this facilitates a policy of selective preoperative CRT for threatened/positive CRM and T4 tumors only. A notable exception is tumors requiring abdominoperineal excision (APE), as unfavorable local recurrence rates necessitate a more aggressive preoperative approach [20].

In the United States, all stage II and III tumors at or below the peritoneal reflection are referred for CRT, increasingly on a preoperative basis. The Swedish and Dutch groups have advocated non-selective SCPRT for all non-metastatic rectal cancers, and this view may be strengthened by the long-term results of CR-07.

Downstaging

"Downstaging" refers to the ability of neoadjuvant therapy to reduce disease stage from that designated at initial assessment to that at final pathological reporting.

This may be interpreted as a simple reduction in T-stage or N-stage alone or as a reduction in AJCC staging [21]. "Downsizing" simply refers to a reduction in tumor volume. The ultimate in downstaging is a pathological complete response (pCR), with no evidence of viable tumor cells.

Sphincter preservation and changing operation

A number of series have reported on the possibility of sphincter preservation following downstaging of low rectal tumors by preoperative therapy initially thought to require APE. These are shown in Table 7.2. Among 194 assigned to APE pre-randomization in CAO/ARO/AIO-94, increased sphincter preservation was possible in the preoperative arm (39% vs. 19%, $p = 0.004$).

Bruce Minsky and colleagues at the Memorial Sloan Kettering Cancer Center presented a series of 27 patients from 1988 to 2003 with T2N0M0 low rectal cancers considered to require APE, but refusing surgery. Preoperative strategy chosen was RT without concomitant chemotherapy, using standard field sizes. Surgery was performed 4–7 weeks later. Sphincter preservation was achieved in 80%. pCR rate was 15%. These patients appear to have comparable local control and survival to matched patients following APE at almost 5 years follow-up.

A contrary outcome is presented in the Polish randomised trial. Surgeons were obliged to base their planned operation on post-RT findings. Disappointingly, there was not a significant difference in sphincter preservation (61% vs. 58%, $p = 0.57$), despite significant downsizing in the long-course arm.

Very careful pathological measurements were presented in this trial. There was an increased distance between tumor and anorectal ring of 1 cm, and a median downsizing of 1.9 cm for the long-course arm. For patients who did undergo low anterior resection, the median distal bowel margin was 2 cm in both arms. This would appear to facilitate sphincter preservation. The authors have postulated that the surgeons violated the rule of choosing operation post-RT because of a bias formed by preoperative review, and a reluctance to change planned operation based on concerns of a positive distal resection margin.

The findings of this trial illustrate a key issue of changing operation. Sphincter preservation following neoadjuvant therapy appears to depend upon philosophy of the surgeon. To some extent, a certain degree of faith in the downstaging and downsizing ability of preoperative CRT is required. The majority of trials to date (see Table 7.2) suggest that sphincter preservation may be achieved safely.

Table 7.2 Randomized-controlled trials of short-course preoperative radiotherapy

RCT	n	Arm A	Arm B	LR	DFS	OS
Swedish Rectal Cancer Trial [12]	1168	Non-selective 25 Gy/5 fractions + surgery	Surgery alone	11% vs. 27% (p < 0.001)	(not provided)	58 vs. 48% (p = 0.004)
Dutch Colorectal Cancer Group [13]	1800	Non-selective 25 Gy/5 fractions + TME	TME alone	2.4% vs. 8.2% (p < 0.001)	(not provided)	82.0% vs. 81.8% (p = 0.84)
Medical Research Council CR-07 [16]	1350	Non-selective 25 Gy/5 fractions + TME	TME alone; PORT for CRM +ve only	3 year: 5% vs. 11% (p < 0.0001) Predicted 5-year: 5% vs. 17%	3 year: 80% vs. 75% (p = 0.03) Predicted 5-year: 75% vs. 67%	3 year: 81% vs. 79% (NS) Predicted 5-year: 72% vs. 62%

RCT = Randomized-controlled trial; PORT = Postoperative radiotherapy;

NS = Non-significant.

Prognostic influence of downstaging

Aside from sphincter preservation, downstaging of rectal cancers appears to hold prognostic significance. At Mount Vernon Cancer Centre, 155 patients with T3 and T4 rectal cancers were treated with preoperative RT with concomitant infusional 5-Fluorouracil [23]. Twelve percent achieved a pCR, and a further 28% were downstaged to T0/1/2. Three-year survival for those achieving downstaging was 64% vs. 25% in those that did not ($p = 0.0001$). Five-year survival in those with R0 resection compared to R1/2 was 70% vs. 30% ($p = 0.02$). Similarly, tumor regression grading (TRG) was evaluated retrospectively for prognostic siginificance upon pathological specimens from the preoperative arm of the German CAO/ARO/A10-94 trail. TRG is a standardized 5-point pathological grading system, grading CRT response from TRG 4, total regression, through grades of fibrosis and residual tumor, to TRG 0, no fibrosis. Five-year disease-free survival following curative resection was 86% for TRG 4, 75% for TRG 2+3, and 63% for TRG 0+1 ($p = 0.006$). The positive impact of downstaging and pCR has been reproduced in other recent series [24,25,26,27], though some have questioned this [28,29]. Non-responders may be considered for more intensive adjuvant chemotherapy.

Interval

There is surprisingly little data to guide clinicians in selecting an appropriate interval from completion of preoperative therapy to surgery. Only one randomized trial exists, the Lyon 90-01, randomizing 201 patients with palpable T2-3 rectal tumors to an interval of 2 weeks vs. 6–8 weeks following neoadjuvant RT [30]. Of note, chemotherapy was not used, and the RT regime was not typical, 39 Gy at 3 Gy per fraction, approximately equivalent to 50 Gy. At a median follow-up of 33 months, there were no significant differences in toxicity, local control, and survival. However, the rate of pathological downstaging (defined here as pCR or "a few residual tumor cells") was 10.3% for a short interval vs. 26% for long ($p = 0.005$).

It is unknown whether a longer interval would facilitate a downstaging effect for SCPRT. This may be answered by an ongoing 3-arm Swedish randomized trial comparing SCPRT with standard short interval, SCPRT and a 6–7 week interval, and long-course 50 Gy over 5 weeks and delayed surgery.

Tumor Bed Boost

As stated, some departments offer a tumor bed boost with external beam RT, to a total dose to gross disease of 50.4–54 Gy. There is no rationale for adding a boost if RT is given for resectable disease. Indeed, one could go so far as to say that in this instance the primary could be blocked and untreated, as it will be fully resected. For irresectable cancers, it is reasonable to add a boost for the purpose of facilitating downsizing, downstaging and complete response, all of which carry prognostic significance.

There is ample evidence of a "dose–response" relationship for local failure, i.e., that higher doses result in further cell kill and a therapeutic gain [6,31]. This relationship is also evidenced by the success of very high dose preoperative endocavitary boost [32]. The Lyon 96-02 trial randomized 90 patients with $T_{2-3}N_0 M_0$ rectal cancers (not involving more than two-third of wall circumference) to preoperative RT 39 Gy in 13 fractions (no concomitant chemotherapy) or the same RT followed by a boost of 85 Gy in 3 fractions delivered with low energy 50 kV "superficial" (i.e., very limited penetration) photons. There was an advantage in favor of the boost arm for complete clinical response at 6 weeks (24% vs. 2%, $p < 0.05$), for pCR (or near-complete, 60.5% vs. 34.9%, $p = 0.027$), and for sphincter preservation (76% vs. 44%, $p = 0.004$). Acute and postoperative toxicity are similar in both arms. The addition of chemotherapy does not seem to enhance the toxicity of this approach [33].

Non-Operative Management

Preoperative treatment for locally advanced rectal cancer has evolved to such a degree that pathological complete response (pCR) rates can reach 25%. This raises the issue as to whether surgery can be avoided for carefully selected patients. To date, only one trial has reported a non-operative strategy for patients achieving a complete response following preoperative CRT, from the University of Sao Paulo [34]. Two hundred and sixty five patients with distal resectable rectal tumors were treated with preoperative CRT from 1991 to 2002. RT was delivered at a dose of 50.4 Gy in 1.8 Gy per fraction for 6 consecutive weeks. Concomitant chemotherapy consisted of 5-Fluorouracil (425 mg/m^2/day) and Leucovorin (20 mg/m^2/day) on the first 3 days and last 3 days of RT. Patients were assessed at 8 weeks (a longer interval than the standard 4–6 weeks) following completion of CRT. Seventy-one patients (26.8%) were judged to have achieved CR on clinical and radiological grounds, though MRI was not used (all patients had preoperative CT, endorectal ultrasound was used in selected cases). These were declared "stage 0" and did not have surgery. All others proceeded to surgery.

At a median follow-up of almost 5-years (57.3 months, range 12–156), overall and disease-free survival rates were 88% and 83% in the resection group and 100% and 92% in the Observation group respectively. Of 71 patients considered to be in "stage 0" following CRT, about 70% were T3, 10% T4, and only 20% radiologically staged as node positive. Twenty percent of patients were T2N0, all of whom were included based upon requirement for APE. Only 2 of these 71 suffered an endoluminal relapse, both of whom were successfully salvaged. Three patients developed metastatic disease.

A pilot study to confirm these findings has commenced at the Royal Marsden Hospital [35].

Acute and chronic toxicity

As survival from rectal cancer continues to improve, with intensive tri-modality therapies, long-term toxicity is being highlighted. Acute RT reactions are defined as those toxicities occurring from the first day of treatment to 30 days post treatment, after which toxicity is considered a "late effect." Factors that influence toxicity include volume irradiated, total dose, dose per fraction, overall treatment time, and technique. Patient-related factors like inflammatory bowel disease (IBD) and previous surgery or radiotherapy may contribute.

Gastro-Intestinal

Acute Gastro-Intestinal (GI) side-effects, such as diarrhea, cramps, tenesmus, proctitis, and the passage of mucus, are experienced by about 80% of patients [36]. In most cases, these symptoms resolve within a few weeks. The pathophysiology of the acute GI inflammatory response to radiotherapy remains poorly understood, though it appears an acute inflammatory response characterized by eosinophilia transforms to a chronic fibrotic response without prominent inflammation. The underlying process is a loss of intestinal crypt mucosal precursor cells. Recovery of the bowel mucosa takes 1–3 months.

Eighty percent of patients will report a permanent change in the behavior of their bowel. Reports of such changes affecting quality of life vary from 6% to 78%. About half of patients will experience diarrhea or constipation. Constipation is a common early effect caused by the physical presence of a rectal mass. Diarrhea as a late effect is multifactorial and thus treatment may need to be appropriated in more than one direction. Serious late effects are uncommon, though some, such as fistulation, sepsis, stenosis, intestinal failure, and transfusion dependent bleeding, may be life threatening. These are estimated to occur in less than 5% after 5–10 years.

The influence of dose per fraction and overall treatment time is illustrated by the SCPRT trials. Fecal incontinence (62% vs. 38% for soiling once a week or less, $p < 0.001$, and 14% vs. 5% for incontinence every day, no p-value given), pad wearing, anal blood and mucus loss, satisfaction with bowel function, and impact of bowel dysfunction on activities of daily living were significantly worse for the SCPRT arm in the Dutch SCPRT trial [37]. Similar results have been described from the Swedish study [38].

The German CAO/ARO/AIO-94 trial displayed a strong trend toward reduced grade III and IV GI effects (chronic diarrhea and small bowel obstruction) in favor of the preoperative arm (9% vs. 15%, $p = 0.07$) [11]. Fecal incontinence rates were not commented upon.

Bladder

Dysuria occurs as an early effect in approximately 20% of patients, though it is generally mild. Infective causes should be outruled. Urinary function did not differ between treatment arms in the Dutch SCPRT trial. Grade III and IV bladder toxicities in CAO/ARO/AIO-94 are quoted at 2% and 4% for the pre- and post-operative arms, respectively ($p = 0.21$).

Reproductive

The testes will generally not receive direct irradiation during RT for rectal cancer. Therefore, exposure is caused by scatter. If a 4-field approach is used, the diverging posterior field contributes about 60% of the scattered dose, and the anterior 30% [39]. A 3-field approach necessitates a higher posterior field weighting, and thus a higher testicular scatter dose. The mean distance of the testicles to the lower field margin has been calculated at between 0.4 cm and 7.2 cm, with a mean of 2.65 cm [39]. Scatter dose to the testes increases exponentially as the distance to the field edge decreases. A testicular shield may reduce the scatter dose by up to 70%–90% [40,41,42].

The testes has been estimated to receive between approximately 0.4 Gy and 3.5 Gy during long-course RT (for a total dose of 50–50.4 Gy) [39,40,43,44].

Clearly, this is dependent on a number of factors, and a boost beyond 45–50 Gy will further escalate dose, although usually such fields have a higher lower border. Germinal epithelium is exquisitely sensitive to low-dose radiation with a negative fractionation effect (i.e., uniquely not affected by fraction size). Recovery is possible, though may take several years, at doses of 1–5 Gy, though in reality greater than 2 Gy is likely to cause permanent azoospermia. However, it is clear that if appropriate technical modifications are made in cases where fertility is at issue, it is likely that testicular dose may be kept below that likely to cause permanent azoospermia, especially for higher tumors.

RT is harmful to both cellular systems of the testis. Leydig cells are less radiosensitive. Nevertheless, a reduction in testosterone levels to about 80% of baseline after pelvic RT is common [39]. This will correspond with a compensatory increase in gonadotropins levels. The extent that this contributes to posttreatment loss of vigor, energy, and sexual function is unknown.

In the female, full-dose pelvic RT will cause sterility in 100%. Ovarian failure shows an age-related radiosensitivity, with doses as low as 2 Gy inducing permanent failure at 45 years, though up to 12 Gy is required for prepubertal females [45]. Like the testes, there is a negative fractionation effect. Shielding or oophoropexy may allow preservation of fertility. Laparoscopic techniques of transposition have become very successful [46].

Embryo cryopreservation is now well established and successful. If a partner is not available, oocyte cryopreservation or vitrification can be performed. Ovarian stimulation is required for this technique and will require a delay in treatment. Immature unstimulated oocytes may be collected and matured and then fertilized and cryopreserved as embryos, or vitrified as mature oocytes. Ovarian tissue cryopreservation remains experimental.

Sexual

There is limited data regarding sexual dysfunction after surgery and/or RT. A series of 18 male bladder Cancer patients of median age 70 at the Western General Hospital, Edinburgh reveals the sexual morbidity of pelvic RT alone on men. No patient had surgery. Each received 52.5 Gy in 20 fractions to the whole bladder with a margin by a conventional 3-field technique. Of 13 (72%) able to achieve an erection prior to RT, 3 became totally impotent 6 months to 5 years after RT. Of the patients retaining potency, about half reported a reduction in the quality of their erections, libido, and frequency of orgasm.

Data for the effect of RT alone on sexual function in women is very limited. A retrospective study of the toxicity of surgery and/or RT for cervical cancer reported little difference in sexual function for RT alone (intracavitary, external beam, or both) compared to surgery alone. Insufficient vaginal lubrication, shortened vagina and insufficient elasticity were significantly higher in women treated with surgery and/or RT compared to matched controls.

The impact of SCPRT on sexual function has been investigated by the Dutch group [47]. About 80% of men and 50% of women were sexually active prior to treatment. Of these, at 24 months, 76% of TME-only men were still active, compared to 67% of those receiving SCPRT + TME ($p = 0.06$); for women, these figures were 90% and 72%, respectively ($p = 0.01$). Male patients experienced erectile and ejaculatory problems, though only the latter was significantly worse in the RT arm ($p = 0.002$). Vaginal dryness and dyspareunia worsened for women, though similarly in both groups. It is interesting to note that overall perceived health did not differ significantly between the two arms.

Secondary malignancy

An analysis of the occurrence of second cancers has recently been published [48] based on the Uppsala trial (completed in 1985, randomly comparing non-selective SCPRT with postoperative RT for stage II and III rectal cancers) [49] and the Swedish SCPRT trial (completed in 1990) [12]. A second cancer was defined as any new cancer other than rectal cancer detected more than 6 months after surgery. Small bowel and colon cancers were excluded. Adenocarcinomas in common sites of metastases within 5 years were not included. The most common second cancers were prostate, colon, and bladder. There were 122 new cancers in 115 patients analyzed. Eight percent of patients in the Uppsala trial and 7% in the Swedish trial developed a second cancer.

More cancers developed in the RT arm of the Swedish trial, reaching significance at 7–8 years ($p = 0.009$). No difference was seen for pre- and postoperative groups in the Uppsala trial. The median interval for the development of a second cancer was 6.5 years (range 1 to 18 years). Interestingly, a trend was seen for an increased risk of malignancy outside the irradiated volume, of almost the same magnitude as for organs within or adjacent. Overall in the Swedish trial, 20.3% of the SCPRT developed either a recurrence or a second cancer, compared to 30.7% of the non-RT patients. This sobering data may encourage a more selective approach to preoperative RT.

Influence of technique on toxicity

A group of 30 patients in the Swedish SCPRT trials were treated with 2 beams, anterior and posterior, a technique associated with increased small bowel irradiation [12]. In-hospital postoperative mortality was 15% (vs. 3% for surgery only, $p < 0.001$). Overall postoperative mortality was similar (4% vs. 3%, $p = 0.3$), as all other patients were treated with a modern multifield technique. A randomized trial by Tait *et al.* of conformal vs. conventional RT for pelvic malignancies ($n = 266$) did not show a symptomatic advantage, despite a reduction in normal tissue irradiation within a "high-dose volume" (792 cm^3 vs. 689 cm^3, $p = 0.02$).

Others

The skin of the abdominal wall is rarely of concern, except in skin folds for obese patients. For patients with low tumors where the perineum is fully treated, acute vaginal and anal erythema and desquamation may be severe, healing with some degree of permanent atrophic and fibrotic change. Long-term toxicities beyond those described, such as pelvic fractures or lumber plexopathy, are rare.

Local excision

Despite advantages in sphincter preservation and operative morbidity and mortality, results of local excision for even T1 rectal tumors have been inferior to radical surgery [50,51]. Trials of adjuvant CRT following local excision have shown encouraging results [52,53], though in keeping with trends in radical surgery, more recent studies have scheduled CRT on a neoadjuvant basis [54,55]. The most exciting and favorable results to date combine neoadjuvant RT with transanal endoscopic microsurgery (TEMS). Lezoche and colleagues enrolled 100 T2/3 node negative rectal adenocarcinomas of diameter < 3 cm, within 8 cm of the anal verge [55]. Preoperative staging included rigid rectoscopy, transanal ultrasound, and MRI or CT. RT was 50.4 Gy at 1.8 Gy per fraction, encompassing the anus, rectum, regional, and iliac lymph nodes. A quarter of patients received continuous infusion 5-Fluorouracil (200 mg/m^2/day).

Patients were restaged 40 days following completion of RT. "Minor" complications occurred in 11 patients, "major" in 2, though symptoms resolved in all patients within 2 months of surgery. At a median follow-up of 55 months, all patients that had tumors downsized (reduced in size $\geq 50\%$) or downstaged (a reduction in T-stage) were free of disease. Cancer-specific survival was 92% for T2 tumors and 85% for T3.

Long-term toxicity and quality of life results are awaited. Longer follow-up is needed to confirm local control. It is hoped that a phase III randomized trial already underway will confirm this promising data. The prospect of response to neoadjuvant therapy dictating radical or local surgery is an enticing one, though local excision is often chosen because of age and/or co-morbidities.

Radiotherapy alone

External beam RT alone for local control is limited by normal tissue toxicity. Delivery of doses higher than 45–50 Gy (small bowel morbidity is unacceptable over this range) is impossible for a large pelvis volume, though higher doses may be given to a reduced field. In modern series, endocavitary irradiation has been used alone [56,57], in conjunction with interstitial brachytherapy [58], or external beam RT, or both [59] to increase tumor dose and thus local control. In general, this strategy is reserved for those unfit for general anesthesia, though avoiding APE may also be an indication. Usually, only a limited circumferential extent or tumor size is eligible.

Despite routine administration of doses in excess of 100 Gy, toxicity is modest. For example, in a series from Jean-Pierre Gerard in Lyon, patients received endocavitary 80 Gy in 3 fractions, then external beam RT 39 Gy in 13 fractions with a 4 Gy boost, and finally 20 Gy via a ^{192}Ir implant [59]. No grade III or IV acute toxicity was seen. Late rectal bleeding occurred in 38%, though only 1 patient required a transfusion. Anorectal function was excellent or good in two-thirds of living patients assessed (Memorial Sloan Kettering Scale). No patient required a colostomy. Results are also remarkable. Local control of over 60%–70% is typical, with T-stage highly prognostic. The above series quotes a 5-year survival of 84% and 53% for T2 and T3 tumors, respectively, for patients < 80 years of age. T1N0 tumors may be treated with endocavitary RT alone, with local control in the region of 85%–90%.

Colon cancer

To our knowledge, no series of neoadjuvant CRT exists for sigmoid or colonic tumors. Willett *et al.* at the Massachusetts General Hospital published the largest retrospective series of adjuvant RT for colonic tumors to date ($n = 203$) [60]. These included patients with colonic T4N0M0 tumors, T3N1-2 in anatomically "immobile" regions (i.e., retroperitoneal), and selected high-risk T3N0 tumors with close margins. Patients were treated with adjuvant RT (45 Gy with a 5-cm margin), without concomitant chemotherapy. Treated patients were compared to a historical group ($n = 395$) treated with surgery only. There was a local control and disease-free survival (DFS) advantage for T4N0M0 (DFS 80%) and T4N + M0 (DFS 53%) tumors, and for T3N0 tumors with a perforation or fistula. There was a 37% 5-year DFS in those having RT following R2 resection (i.e., gross disease left *in situ*). Ten-year results confirm these outcomes, especially in the T4N0 subset.

Intergroup-0130 was developed based on Willett's data [61]. This trial was abandoned owing to poor accrual; only 222 of an anticipated 400 patients were recruited, 34 patients proving ineligible. Eligible patients had T4 or selected T3N1-2 resected colonic neoplasms. Randomization was 12 cycles of bolus 5-FU and Levamisole with or without RT (45–50.4 Gy), starting at cycle 2. Again toxicity was acceptable, though there was no significant survival or disease-free survival advantage.

While it does seem reasonable to treat certain high-risk colonic tumors with adjuvant therapy, there is little doubt that the evidence-base for adjuvant RT or CRT for sigmoid and colonic tumors is less certain than that for true rectal cancers, and there is no body of neoadjuvant evidence.

Hepatic radiotherapy

Although the development of liver metastases from colorectal carcinoma has traditionally heralded a very poor prognosis, the advent of more efficacious systemic therapy has improved median survival from months to years. Hepatic metastasectomy may improve long-term survival in selected patients, but curative resection is feasible in less than 25% of patients [62]. Radiofrequency ablation is an established technique, but may not treat tumors > 5 cm, or abutting vasculature or bile ducts. Thus, many patients with unresectable disease limited to the liver are unsuitable for other local therapies.

Although whole liver hepatic irradiation has resulted in significant symptomatic palliation [63,64,65,66], no clear survival benefit has been demonstrated. Hepatic irradiation has evolved into the delivery of tumoricidal doses to partial liver volumes beyond the typical 20–30 Gy to the whole liver. Trials of 3D conformal RT have demonstrated the safe irradiation of focal hepatic malignancies to much higher doses while sparing significant portions of the normal liver, and have suggested a survival advantage [67,68,69].

A recent phase II trial delivered focal hepatic RT with intra-arterial floxuridine to 128 patients with primary hepatobiliary cancers or colorectal metastases [70]. The prescribed dose was dependent upon the risk of induction of radiation-induced liver disease, ranging from 40 Gy to 90 Gy (median 60.75 Gy). RT was administered in two

2-week blocks with a 2-week gap. 1.5 Gy was delivered twice-daily five days a week and once on Saturdays. Median survival for colorectal patients was 17.2 months. Furthermore, the only predictor of survival was the dose of radiation given. Median survival for those receiving less than 60.7 Gy was 15.2 months (95% CI, 9.5–16.4 months), while that of patients receiving more was 18.4 months (95% CI, 12.9–22.8 months). Thirty percent developed grade III or IV toxicities, the most common being upper GI ulceration and bleeding, radiation-induced liver disease and catheter-related problems. One patient died as a result of treatment.

Radiotherapy for locally recurrent disease

Patients that are RT-naïve with localized failure only may of course be safely administered preoperative CRT for resectable or irresectable disease. Data of outcome of surgical salvage following RT is limited, though supportive of tri-modality therapy [71]. Re-irradiation is associated with enhanced toxicity. At the University of Kentucky, 103 patients with recurrent rectal adenocarcinoma were re-irradiated with concurrent 5-Fluorouracil [72]. Of these, 34 were referred for surgery (5-year survival 22%). Median cumulative dose was 85.8 Gy (range 70–100 Gy). Volumes were small, centered around gross disease and excluding bladder and small bowel.

Twenty-two percent required a treatment break or early cessation of CRT for diarrhea or perineal skin breakdown. Fifteen percent developed small bowel obstruction as a late complication, though most responded to conservative measures. No patient suffered anastomotic or delayed wound dehiscence, soft tissue necrosis, or overt bone fractures. Longer interval to re-irradiation was associated with a reduction in late toxicity.

REFERENCES

1. Gunderson, L. L. and Sosin, H. Areas of failure found at reoperation (second or symptomatic look) following "curative surgery" for adenocarcinoma of the rectum. Clinicopathologic correlation and implications for adjuvant therapy. *Cancer* **34** (1974), 1278–92.
2. Wiig, J. N., Wolff, P. A., Tveit, K. M., *et al.* Location of pelvic recurrence after 'curative' low anterior resection for rectal cancer. *Eur J Surg Oncol*, **25** (1999), 590–4.
3. Hruby, G., Barton, M., Miles, S., *et al.* Sites of local recurrence after surgery, with or without chemotherapy, for rectal cancer: implications for radiotherapy field design. *Int J Radiat Oncol Biol Phys*, **55** (2003), 138–43.

4. Steup, W. H., Moriya, Y., and van de Velde, C. J. Patterns of lymphatic spread in rectal cancer. A topographical analysis on lymph node metastases. *Eur J Cancer*, **38** (2002), 911–18.

5. Hocht, S., Hammad, R., Thiel, H. J., *et al.* Recurrent rectal cancer within the pelvis. A multicenter analysis of 123 patients and recommendations for adjuvant radiotherapy. *Strahlenther Onkol*, **180** (2004), 15–20.

6. Fisher, B., Wolmark, N., Rockette, H., *et al.* Postoperative adjuvant chemotherapy or radiation therapy for rectal cancer: results from NSABP protocol R-01. *J Natl Cancer Inst*, **80** (1988), 21–9.

7. Randomised trial of surgery alone versus surgery followed by radiotherapy for mobile cancer of the rectum. Medical Research Council Rectal Cancer Working Party. *Lancet*, **348** (1996), 1610–14.

8. Prolongation of the disease-free interval in surgically treated rectal carcinoma. Gastrointestinal Tumor Study Group. *N Engl J Med* **312** (1985), 1465–72.

9. Wolmark, N., Wieand, H. S., Hyams, D. M., *et al.* Randomized trial of postoperative adjuvant chemotherapy with or without radiotherapy for carcinoma of the rectum: National Surgical Adjuvant Breast and Bowel Project Protocol R-02. *J Natl Cancer Inst*, **92** (2000), 388–96.

10. Roh, M., Petrelli, N., Wieand, S., *et al.* Phase III randomized trial of preoperative versus postoperative mutimodality therapy in patients with carcinoma of the rectum (NSABPR-03). *2001 ASCO General Meeting* (2005), abstr 490.

11. Sauer, R., Becker, H., Hohenberger, W., *et al.* Preoperative versus postoperative chemoradiotherapy for rectal cancer. *N Engl J Med*, **351** (2004), 1731–40.

12. Improved survival with preoperative radiotherapy in resectable rectal cancer. Swedish Rectal Cancer Trial. *N Engl J Med*, **336** (1997), 980–7.

13. Kapiteijn, E., Marijnen, C. A., Nagtegaal, I. D., *et al.* Preoperative radiotherapy combined with total mesorectal excision for resectable rectal cancer. *N Engl J Med*, **345** (2001), 638–46.

14. Marijnen, C. A., Nagtegaal, I. D., Kapiteijn, E., *et al.* Radiotherapy does not compensate for positive resection margins in rectal cancer patients: report of a multicenter randomized trial. *Int J Radiat Oncol Biol Phys*, **55** (2003), 1311–20.

15. Bosset, J. F., Calais, G., Mineur, L., *et al.* Enhanced tumorocidal effect of chemotherapy with preoperative radiotherapy for rectal cancer: preliminary results – EORTC 22921. *J Clin Oncol*, **23** (2005), 5620–7.

16. Sebag-Montefiore, D., Steele, R., Quirke, P., *et al.* Routine short course pre-op radiotherapy or selective post-op chemoradiotherapy for resectable rectal cancer? Preliminary results of the MRC CR07 randomised trial. *J Clin Oncol (Meeting Abstracts)*, **24** (2006), 3511 [Abstract].

17. Nagtegaal, I. D., van de Velde, C. J., van der Worp, E., *et al.* Macroscopic evaluation of rectal cancer resection specimen: clinical significance of the pathologist in quality control. *J Clin Oncol*, **20** (2002), 1729–34.

18. Bujko, K., Nowacki, M. P., Nasierowska-Guttmejer, A., *et al.* Long-term results of a randomized trial comparing preoperative short-course radiotherapy with preoperative conventionally fractionated chemoradiation for rectal cancer. *Br J Surg*, **93** (2006), 1215–23.

19. Diagnostic accuracy of preoperative magnetic resonance imaging in predicting curative resection of rectal cancer: prospective observational study. *Bmj,* **333** (2006), 779.

20. Marr, R., Birbeck, K., Garvican, J., *et al.* The modern abdominoperineal excision: the next challenge after total mesorectal excision. *Ann Surg,* **242** (2005), 74–82.

21. *AJCC Cancer Staging Handbook Sixth edition* (American Joint Committee on Cancer, 2002).

22. Bujko, K., Nowacki, M. P., Nasierowska-Guttmejer, A., *et al.* Sphincter preservation following preoperative radiotherapy for rectal cancer: report of a randomised trial comparing short-term radiotherapy vs. conventionally fractionated radiochemotherapy. *Radiother Oncol* **72** (2004), 15–24.

23. Mawdsley, S. and Glynne-Jones, R. The importance of pathological downstaging and the circumferential margin in rectal carcinomas treated with neoadjuvant chemoradiation. *ASCO Annual Meeting,* (2005), abstr 3642.

24. Balch, G. C., Mithani, S. K., Shyr, Y., *et al.* Prognostic significance of response to neoadjuvant chemoradiation therapy for rectal cancer. *ASCO Annual Meeting* (2003), abstr 1047.

25. Shivnani, T., Small, W., Stryker, S. J., *et al.* Preoperative chemoradiation in Rectal Cancer: correlation of tumor response with survival. *J Clin Oncol Proc* (2004), abstr 247.

26. Rodel, C., Martus, P., Papadoupolos, T., *et al.* Prognostic significance of tumor regression after preoperative chemoradiotherapy for rectal cancer. *J Clin Oncol,* **23** (2005), 8688–96.

27. Vecchio, F. M., Valentini, V., Minsky, B. D., *et al.* The relationship of pathologic tumor regression grade (TRG) and outcomes after preoperative therapy in rectal cancer. *Int J Radiat Oncol Biol Phys,* **62** (2005), 752–60.

28. Pucciarelli, S., Toppan, P., Friso, M. L., *et al.* Complete pathologic response following preoperative chemoradiation therapy for middle to lower rectal cancer is not a prognostic factor for a better outcome. *Dis Colon Rectum,* **47** (2004), 1798–807.

29. Glynne-Jones, R. and Anyamene, N. Just how useful an endpoint is complete pathological response after neoadjuvant chemoradiation in rectal cancer? *Int J Radiat Oncol Biol Phys,* **66** (2006), 319–20.

30. Francois, Y., Nemoz, C. J., Baulieux, J., *et al.* Influence of the interval between preoperative radiation therapy and surgery on downstaging and on the rate of sphincter-sparing surgery for rectal cancer: the Lyon R90–01 randomized trial. *J Clin Oncol,* **17** (1999), 2396.

31. Goldberg, P. A., Nicholls, R. J., Porter, N. H., *et al.* Long-term results of a randomised trial of short-course low-dose adjuvant pre-operative radiotherapy for rectal cancer: reduction in local treatment failure. *Eur J Cancer,* **30A** (1994), 1602–6.

32. Gerard, J. P., Chapet, O., Nemoz, C., *et al.* Improved sphincter preservation in low rectal cancer with high-dose preoperative radiotherapy: the lyon R96–02 randomized trial. *J Clin Oncol,* **22** (2004), 2404–9.

33. Jakobsen, A., Mortensen, J. P., Bisgaard, C., *et al.* Preoperative chemoradiation of locally advanced T3 rectal cancer combined with an endorectal boost. *Int J Radiat Oncol Biol Phys,* **64** (2006), 461–5.

34. *J clin Oncol,* **23** (2005), 8688–96.

35. *Lancet Oncol,* **8** (2007), 625–33.

36. Andreyev, J. Gastrointestinal complications of pelvic radiotherapy: are they of any importance? *Gut*, **54** (2005), 1051–4.

37. Peeters, K. C., van de Velde, C. J., Leer, J. W., *et al.* Late side effects of short-course preoperative radiotherapy combined with total mesorectal excision for rectal cancer: increased bowel dysfunction in irradiated patients – a Dutch colorectal cancer group study. *J Clin Oncol*, **23** (2005), 199–206.

38. Dahlberg, M., Glimelius, B., Graf, W., *et al.* Preoperative irradiation affects functional results after surgery for rectal cancer: results from a randomized study. *Dis Colon Rectum*, **41** (1998), 543–9, discussion 549–51.

39. Hermann, R. M., Henkel, K., Christiansen, H., *et al.* Testicular dose and hormonal changes after radiotherapy of rectal cancer. *Radiother Oncol* **75** (2005), 83–8.

40. Mazonakis, M., Damilakis, J., Varveris, H., *et al.* Radiation dose to testes and risk of infertility from radiotherapy for rectal cancer. *Oncol Rep* **15** (2006), 729–33.

41. Fraass, B. A., Kinsella, T. J., Harrington, F. S., *et al.* Peripheral dose to the testes: the design and clinical use of a practical and effective gonadal shield. *Int J Radiat Oncol Biol Phys*, **11** (1985), 609–15.

42. Kubo, H. and Shipley, W. U. Reduction of the scatter dose to the testicle outside the radiation treatment fields. *Int J Radiat Oncol Biol Phys*, **8** (1982), 1741–5.

43. Budgell, G. J., Cowan, R. A., and Hounsell, A. R. Prediction of scattered dose to the testes in abdominopelvic radiotherapy. *Clin Oncol (R Coll Radiol)*, **13** (2001), 120–5.

44. Piroth, M. D., Hensley, F., Wannenmacher, M., *et al.* [Male gonadal dose in adjuvant 3-d-pelvic irradiation after anterior resection of rectal cancer. Influence to fertility]. *Strahlenther Onkol*, **179** (2003), 754–9.

45. Spinelli, S., Chiodi, S., Bacigalupo, A., *et al.* Ovarian recovery after total body irradiation and allogeneic bone marrow transplantation: long-term follow up of 79 females. *Bone Marrow Transplant*, **14** (1994), 373–80.

46. Bisharah, M. and Tulandi, T. Laparoscopic preservation of ovarian function: an underused procedure. *Am J Obstet Gynecol*, **188** (2003), 367–70.

47. Marijnen, C. A., van de Velde, C. J., Putter, H., *et al.* Impact of short-term preoperative radiotherapy on health-related quality of life and sexual functioning in primary rectal cancer: report of a multicenter randomized trial. *J Clin Oncol*, **23** (2005), 1847–58.

48. Birgisson, H., Pahlman, L., Gunnarsson, U., *et al.* Occurrence of second cancers in patients treated with radiotherapy for rectal cancer. *J Clin Oncol*, **23** (2005), 6126–31.

49. Frykholm, G. J., Glimelius, B., and Pahlman, L. Preoperative or postoperative irradiation in adenocarcinoma of the rectum: final treatment results of a randomized trial and an evaluation of late secondary effects. *Dis Colon Rectum*, **36** (1993), 564–72.

50. Bentrem, D. J., Okabe, S., Wong, W. D., *et al.* T1 adenocarcinoma of the rectum: transanal excision or radical surgery? *Ann Surg*, **242** (2005), 472–7, discussion 477–9.

51. You, Y. N., Baxter, N., Stewart, A., *et al.* Is local excision adequate for T1 rectal cancer? A nationwide cohort study from the national cancer database (NCDB). *ASCO Annual Meeting*, (2005), abstr 3526.

52. Steele, G. D. Jr., Herndon, J. E., Bleday, R., *et al*. Sphincter-sparing treatment for distal rectal adenocarcinoma. *Ann Surg Oncol*, **6** (1996), 433–41.

53. Russell, A. H., Harris, J., Rosenberg, P. J., *et al*. Anal sphincter conservation for patients with adenocarcinoma of the distal rectum: long-term results of radiation therapy oncology group protocol 89–02. *Int J Radiat Oncol Biol Phys*, **46** (2000), 313–22.

54. Kim, C. J., Yeatman, T. J., Coppola, D., *et al*. Local excision of T2 and T3 rectal cancers after downstaging chemoradiation. *Ann Surg*, **234** (2001), 352–8, discussion 358–9.

55. Lezoche, E., Guerrieri, M., Paganini, A. M., *et al*. Long-term results in patients with T2-3 N0 distal rectal cancer undergoing radiotherapy before transanal endoscopic microsurgery. *Br J Surg*, **92** (2005), 1546–52.

56. Gerard, J. P., Ayzac, L., Coquard, R., *et al*. Endocavitary irradiation for early rectal carcinomas T1 (T2). A series of 101 patients treated with the Papillon's technique. *Int J Radiat Oncol Biol Phys*, **34** (1996), 775–83.

57. Lavertu, S., Schild, S. E., Gunderson, L. L., *et al*. Endocavitary radiation therapy for rectal adenocarcinoma: 10-year results. *Am J Clin Oncol*, **26** (2003), 508–12.

58. Coatmeur, O., Truc, G., Barillot, I., *et al*. Treatment of T1-T2 rectal tumors by contact therapy and interstitial brachytherapy. *Radiother Oncol*, **70** (2004), 177–82.

59. Gerard, J. P., Chapet, O., Ramaioli, A., *et al*. Long-term control of T2-T3 rectal adenocarcinoma with radiotherapy alone. *Int J Radiat Oncol Biol Phys*, **54** (2002), 142–9.

60. Willett, C. G., Fung, C. Y., Kaufman, D. S., *et al*. Postoperative radiation therapy for high-risk colon carcinoma. *J Clin Oncol*, **11** (1993), 1112–17.

61. Martenson, J. A., Jr., Willett, C. G., Sargent, D. J., *et al*. Phase III study of adjuvant chemotherapy and radiation therapy compared with chemotherapy alone in the surgical adjuvant treatment of colon cancer: results of intergroup protocol 0130. *J Clin Oncol*, **22** (2004), 3277–83.

62. Adson, M. A. Resection of liver metastases – when is it worthwhile? *World J Surg*, **11** (1987), 511–20.

63. Borgelt, B. B., Gelber, R., Brady, L. W., *et al*. The palliation of hepatic metastases: results of the Radiation Therapy Oncology Group pilot study. *Int J Radiat Oncol Biol Phys*, **7** (1981), 587–91.

64. Phillips, R., Karnofsky, D. A., Hamilton, L. D., *et al*. Roentgen therapy of hepatic metastases. *Am J Roentgenol Radium Ther Nucl Med*, **71** (1954), 826–34.

65. Prasad, B., Lee, M. S., and Hendrickson, F. R. Irradiation of hepatic metastases. *Int J Radiat Oncol Biol Phys*, **2** (1977), 129–32.

66. Sherman, D. M., Weichselbaum, R., Order, S. E., *et al*. Palliation of hepatic metastasis. *Cancer*, **41** (1978), 2013–17.

67. Robertson, J. M., Lawrence, T. S., Walker, S., *et al*. The treatment of colorectal liver metastases with conformal radiation therapy and regional chemotherapy. *Int J Radiat Oncol Biol Phys*, **32** (1995), 445–50.

68. Jackson, A., Ten Haken, R. K., Robertson, J. M., *et al*. Analysis of clinical complication data for radiation hepatitis using a parallel architecture model. *Int J Radiat Oncol Biol Phys*, **31** (1995), 883–91.

69. Dawson, L. A., McGinn, C. J., Normolle, D., *et al.* Escalated focal liver radiation and concurrent hepatic artery fluorodeoxyuridine for unresectable intrahepatic malignancies. *J Clin Oncol*, **18** (2000), 2210–18.

70. Ben-Josef, E., Normolle, D., Ensminger, W. D., *et al.* Phase II trial of high-dose conformal radiation therapy with concurrent hepatic artery floxuridine for unresectable intrahepatic malignancies. *J Clin Oncol*, **23** (2005), 8739–47.

71. Vermaas, M., Ferenschild, F. T., Nuyttens, J. J., *et al.* Preoperative radiotherapy improves outcome in recurrent rectal cancer. *Dis Colon Rectum*, **48** (2005), 918–28.

72. Mohiuddin, M., Marks, G., and Marks, J. Long-term results of reirradiation for patients with recurrent rectal carcinoma. *Cancer*, **95** (2002), 1144–50.

8

The changing role of endoluminal ultrasound in rectal cancer

Peter Chowdhury, Rhodri Davies, and Ashley Roberts

Introduction

Modern-day management of rectal carcinoma should take place within a multi-disciplinary setting and precise imaging retains a pivotal role. The fundamental purpose of imaging is to predict the pathological stage, allowing patients who require neoadjuvant therapy to be identified while preventing those with early rectal cancers from unnecessary treatment.

The aim of neoadjuvant therapy is to reduce the risk of local recurrence following "curative" surgery which has a reported incidence of 3%–32% [1]. It has been shown that such treatment is more effective if given preoperatively [2,3] and the latest results from the Swedish rectal cancer trial have reported long-term survival benefits as well as a reduction in local recurrence between the irradiated and non-irradiated group (9% vs. 26%) [4].

Preoperative staging of rectal cancer presents a challenge to radiologists and endoscopists alike. The available imaging modalities include CT, MRI and endoluminal ultrasound [5]. Endoscopists, on the other hand, are entering a new era of direct mucosal imaging by means of magnifying chromoendoscopy [6], a technique with which most radiologists are unfamiliar.

Despite recent technological advances, the current role of CT is largely for detecting distant metastases although local tumor staging is possible [7,8,9] and widely practiced [10]. The main drawbacks are its inability to resolve the different layers of the rectal wall and reliably determine the presence of lymph node metastases.

In recent years, MRI has become the preferred imaging modality in patients with more advanced rectal cancer [11,12]. MRI has better contrast resolution than CT and is able to resolve different layers of the rectal wall, and perhaps of greater significance, MRI demonstrates the mesorectal fascia. Involvement of this fascial plane means the surgeon may not achieve a clear circumferential resection margin (CRM) at the time of total mesorectal excision (TME) [13]. Brown *et al.* [14] suggest MRI can predict CRM positive status when tumor is imaged to within 1 mm of the mesorectal fascia.

MRI has thus revolutionized the management of more advanced rectal cancer by distinguishing those who are likely to benefit from neoadjuvant therapy (anticipated close or involved margin at TME) from those who are not.

It is against this background that the future role of endorectal ultrasound (ERUS) has to be redefined. One promising application is the assessment of early disease that is at low risk for lymph node metastases and potentially curable by local excision alone.

Anatomy, equipment, and techniques

Wild and Reid first used intraluminal ultrasound to image the rectum in the late 1950s [15]. By the early 1980s, ultrasound technology had improved sufficiently to permit its use as a clinical tool in rectal cancer staging [16,17]. At first, it was possible to resolve two or three layers of the rectal wall [18,19]. Later work by Beynon *et al.* [20] using 7 MHz transducers described the rectal wall as having five sonographic layers (Figure 8.1):
1. Interface between water-filled balloon and superficial mucosa (hyperechoic)
2. Deep mucosa (hypoechoic)

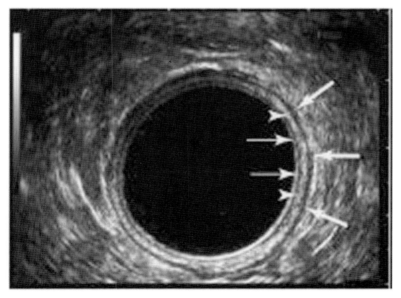

Figure 8.1   ERUS of normal rectal wall. Deep mucosa = innermost hypoechoic band (thin arrow); submucosa = hyperechoic band (arrowhead); muscularis propria = outermost hypoechoic band (thick arrow).

3. Submucosa (hyperechoic)
4. Muscularis propria (hypoechoic)
5. Perirectal tissues (hyperechoic).

While the resolution of the rectal wall into these layers is unsurpassed by other imaging techniques, the main disadvantage of ERUS is the inability to directly image the mesorectal fascia. The relationship of this to the primary tumor plays a critical role in preoperative staging of advanced cancer and is well demonstrated by MRI. Given these advantages and disadvantages, it is therefore almost inevitable that the role of ERUS will gravitate to earlier disease.

A variety of endoluminal ultrasound instruments are available: rigid probes, flexible echoendoscopes, and more recently miniprobes. Radial devices are the most widely used, and produce a 360-degree image perpendicular to the long axis of the instrument. However, in certain situations, a linear echoendoscope may be used to permit fine needle aspiration (FNA) of suspicious lesions (e.g., regional lymphadenopathy) [21,22,23,24]. Here, the scan plane is parallel to the endoscope axis so when a needle is passed out of the biopsy channel, its tip can be accurately advanced into the target lesion (Figure 8.2 A–D).

Rigid probes are limited by their inability to traverse stenotic tumors and up to 17% may be impossible to stage [25]. It may also be difficult to reach the upper

(A)

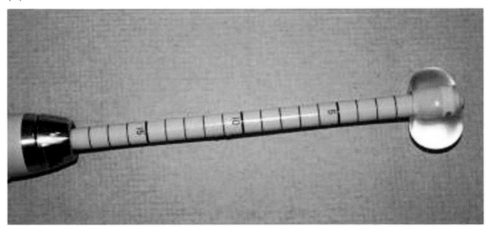

Figure 8.2   (A) Rigid Hitachi probe with rectal balloon filled with water for acoustic coupling. (B) Tip of the Olympus UM 2000 radial echoendoscope. (C) Tip of the Olympus GFUCT 240 electronic linear array echoendoscope. A needle has been passed into the biopsy channel. (D) A Fujinon 20-MHz miniprobe exiting the biopsy channel of a flexible sigmoidoscope.

(B)

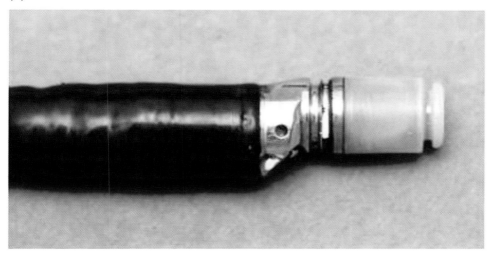

(C)

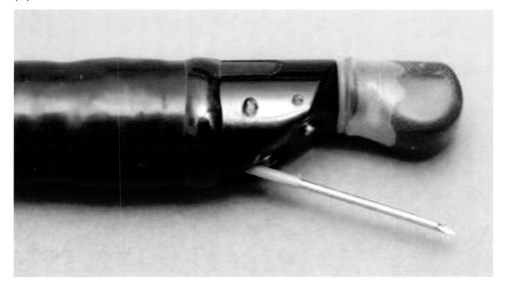

Figure 8.2   (cont.)

rectum, and keep the ultrasound beam perpendicular to the mucosa. Scanning the mucosa at an oblique angle can lead to inaccurate staging as the rectal wall layers appear spuriously thickened. These problems may be overcome by miniprobes, which are passed down the biopsy channel at the time of endoscopy, or flexible

(D)

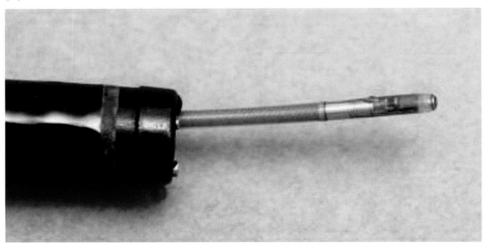

Figure 8.2   (cont.)

echoendoscopes [26]. However, these systems are more complex, expensive, and less widely available than rigid probes.

Staging accuracy of ERUS

Promising results for ERUS have been reported with T-stage accuracy up to 96% [27] although performance may be overestimated in the literature owing to publication bias [28]. Nonetheless, by assessing tumor penetration (hypoechoic mass lesion) in relation to the rectal wall layers, it is possible to provide an ultrasound T stage which correlates well with the T component of the TNM classification (Figures 8.3 and 8.4):

1. uT1: tumor confined to mucosa and submucosa
2. uT2: tumor confined to rectal wall (i.e., involves muscularis propria)
3. uT3: tumor extends through rectal wall into perirectal fat (i.e., beyond muscularis propria)
4. uT4: tumor invades surrounding organs

Overstaging of T2 lesions is well described and is caused by peritumoral inflammation merging imperceptibly with the primary tumor [25,29,30]. A possible consequence (although practices vary from country to country) is unnecessary radiotherapy and hence potential related morbidity. Overstaging can also occur with oblique scanning as mentioned above, and over-distension of the coupling

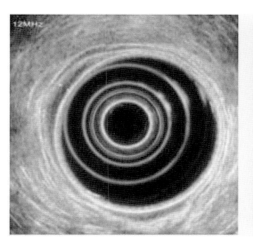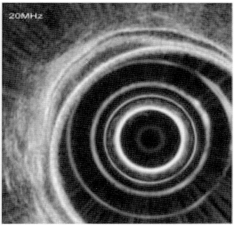

Figure 8.3   The effect of increasing frequency on image resolution. By increasing the frequency from 12 MHz to 20 MHz, the resolution of this subtle lesion confined to the mucosa (T1) is improved (caliper markers).

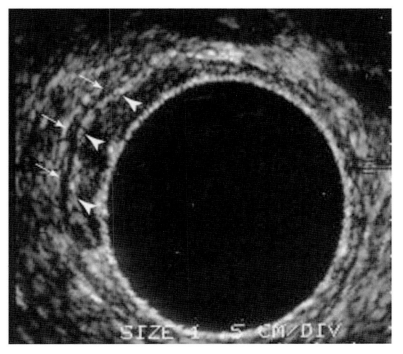

Figure 8.4   Superficial rectal tumor confined to mucosa (T1). Note the intact hyperechoic submucosa (arrowheads) medial to the muscularis propria (arrows). This was a moderately dysplastic tubulovillous adenoma on histopathology.

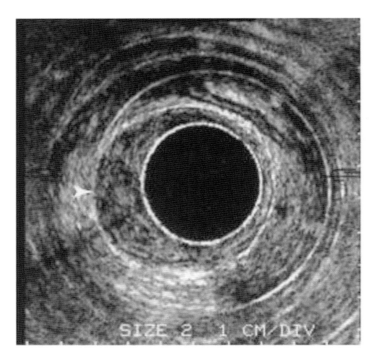

Figure 8.5 Over-distension of the coupling balloon has made the muscularis propria indistinct in the 9 o'clock position (arrowhead). This lesion was thought to be T2 on ERUS but was in fact confined to the mucosa on histopathology (pT1).

balloon (Figure 8.5). Conversely, understaging occurs less commonly, and is the result of microscopic tumor infiltration below the resolution capabilities of ultrasound (Figure 8.6).

The assessment of lymph nodes is less accurate than T staging with accuracies ranging between 64% and 83% [27]. While size greater than 1 cm, hypoechoic texture, distinct margins, and round shape can suggest malignant involvement, none of these features are consistently reliable. Such nodes could be targeted by ERUS-FNA if clinically relevant [31] to obtain samples for cytological examination and/or methylation analysis for the detection of lymph node micrometastases [32]. Some authors believe that the mere visualization alone of perirectal lymph nodes is evidence enough of involvement since non-metastatic nodes are typically not seen on ERUS [33]. Others have shown that a negative ERUS–FNA will effect a change in management in a significant proportion of patients by downstaging their disease and hence avoiding unnecessary neoadjuvant therapy [34]. We have some concerns ERUS–FNA could potentially convert N0 disease into N1 disease if involved mucosa is traversed by the needle.

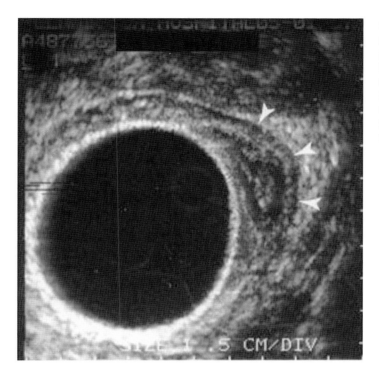

Figure 8.6   The muscularis propria (arrowheads) appears intact on ERUS suggesting this is a T1 lesion. Histopathology revealed tumor cells infiltrating the muscle coat (pT2).

Potential impact of ERUS on early rectal cancer management: beyond TNM

ERUS has largely been concerned with providing a preoperative stage according to the TNM classification as outlined earlier. However, with early disease (T1), further classifications are required beyond the TNM system. T1 tumors must therefore be sub-classified, as a clear relationship exists between the depth of tumor penetration and the likelihood of lymph node metastasis [35,36,37] as well as local recurrence [38,39].

Haggitt's classification of early colorectal carcinoma has been in use since 1985 and describes 4 levels of invasion in a pedunculated adenoma [40] (Figure 8.7). Again the central principle is that the depth of invasion is the major factor in determining prognosis. Pedunculated adenomas by nature of their stalk provide a greater distance over which an invasive carcinoma has to traverse before reaching the submucosa of the underlying bowel wall (Haggitt level 4). These lesions in addition to sessile lesions with submucosal invasion (also Haggitt level 4) have a risk of lymph node metastasis of approx 10% whereas the more superficial lesions (Haggitt level 1, 2, or 3) have a low risk of metastasis [41].

The Japanese have further classified sessile T1 lesions by subdividing the submucosa into thirds: sm1, 2, and 3 (superficial, middle, and deep thirds,

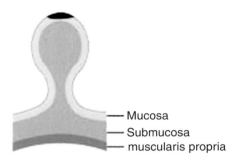

Level 0: non-invasive carcinoma *in situ*

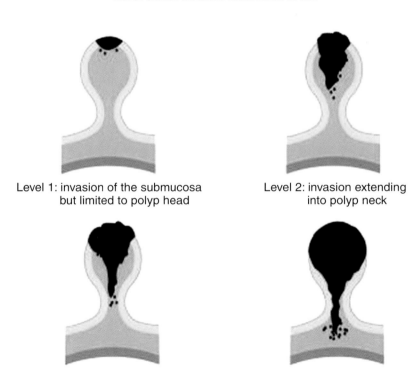

Level 1: invasion of the submucosa   Level 2: invasion extending
but limited to polyp head   into polyp neck

Level 3: invasion into any part of the stalk   Level 4: Invasion beyond the stalk but
                                                              above the muscularis propria

Figure 8.7   Haggitt's classification of early colorectal carcinoma in polyps.

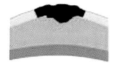
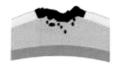
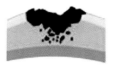

Sm1
Invasion to a depth
of 200–300 µm

Sm2
Intermediate
between Sm1 and Sm3

Sm3
Carcinoma invasion
near to the
muscularis propria

Figure 8.8   Vertical invasion of the submucosa in a sessile lesion.

respectively) [42,43] (Figure 8.8). These authors have found that not all sessile polyps with submucosal invasion are associated with the same risk (cf. Haggitt who classed all such lesions as level 4).

The risk of lymph node metastases is very low for cancers limited to the mucosa and upper third of the submucosa (sm1) [42,43,44,45]. With sm2 involvement, there is a substantially higher risk of lymph node metastases of between 5% and 10% [46]. Akasu and colleagues [45] found that for massive submucosal invasion which they defined as sm2 or sm3, the incidence rises to around 25%.

Thus, a subgroup of patients exists ($\leq$ sm1 disease) who can be treated with curative intent by a variety of minimally invasive means including endoscopic polypectomy and endoscopic mucosal resection (EMR). In the Kikuchi study [43], of 105 patients with sessile-type polyps, 32 were classed as sm1. None of this group showed lymph node metastasis or local recurrence after at least 5-year follow-up.

An ideal staging strategy should be capable of imaging the leading edge of invasive carcinoma so that its depth within the submucosa can be accurately assessed. Whether or not high frequency miniprobe ERUS (m-ERUS) can play a significant diagnostic role in this regard remains unclear.

Workers evaluating a 15-MHz miniprobe [47] found disappointing accuracy (37.1%) when trying to assess the degree of submucosal invasion into the 3 subclasses (sm1, 2, and 3). However, discriminating between $\leq$ sm1 (m and sm1) and $\geq$ sm2 (sm2, 3, muscularis propria, and serosa), a high degree of accuracy was achieved (85.7%). The authors stressed the importance of this differentiation in deciding which patients would be suitable for EMR. Such therapy on deeply invasive lesions ($\geq$ sm2) could result in increased morbidity and require subsequent radical curative surgery.

A frequently quoted advantage of m-ERUS is its ability to cross stenotic lesions. Such lesions in the rectum are unlikely to reflect early disease and hence this advantage may not be relevant. Furthermore, it is difficult to detect pericolic lymph node metastases using m-ERUS because of limited depth of penetration. However, as resolution is improved, it is possible that high-frequency probes will hold the key to staging these early tumors beyond the TNM classification.

Other techniques for assessing tumor stage: endoscopic evaluation

ERUS is not the only means by which early rectal cancer can be assessed. Advances in endoscopic technology and the use of endoscopic dyes can enhance diagnostic information gained by direct visualization.

Flat- and depressed-type colorectal lesions have been recognized for some time by Japanese endoscopists following their initial description by Muto [48]. Recent studies have shown that they are also prevalent in Western cohorts [49,50,51,52,53] although most flat/depressed carcinomas are located in the right colon [52]. Such lesions are more prone to invade the submucosa compared to pedunculated lesions.

A morphological classification of early colorectal lesions from the Japanese Research Society is illustrated in Table 8.1 [54,55]. Neoplastic lesions that appear superficial at endoscopy are classified as subtypes of "type 0" [56]. Submucosal invasion is rare in polypoid lesions less than 1 cm in diameter but increases in proportion to size. Sessile lesions (0 – Is) are more likely to show submucosal invasion than pedunculated polyps (0 – Ip). Depressed lesions of all types (0 – IIc; IIa + IIc; IIc + IIa) show much higher rates of submucosal invasion even if the diameter is less than 1 cm [55,56].

The conspicuity of flat/depressed lesions can be increased by a combination of endoscopic dyes, e.g., indigo carmine (0.2%–1.0%), and high magnification endoscopy capable of magnifying the object image up to 100 times, e.g., Olympus C240Z colonoscope. This allows for a very detailed view of the mucosal surface and clearer representation of surface pit patterns. The Kudo criteria [57] for classifying pit patterns is shown in Table 8.2.

Broadly speaking, pit patterns can be subdivided into neoplastic (IIIL, IV, IIIs, V(a/n)) and non-neoplastic (I, II) classes. Those associated with early invasive colorectal cancer are Types IIIs and V. Type IIIs pits are small round pits often seen in depressed type lesions with high risk of submucosal invasion. Type V pits, also associated with invasion, can be further subdivided into Va type which shows an irregular or random pattern of pit structures and Vn where there is no discernable pit pattern (Figure 8.9).

Table 8.1 Morphological classification of early colorectal lesions from the Japanese Research Society

Endoscopic appearance	Classification		Description
Protruding	0-Ip		Pedunculated
	0-Is		Sessile
Non-protruding and non-excavated	0-IIa		Slightly elevated
	0-IIb		Completely flat
	0-IIc		Slightly depressed
Elevation plus depression	0-IIc + IIa		Depressed lesion with elevation in part of peripheral ring
	0-IIa + IIc		Elevated lesion with central depression

Flat/depressed lesions showing type V pit pattern are likely to be sm2 or sm3 lesions. A recent study evaluating the accuracy of predicting submucosal invasion from identification of type V pits using high magnification chromoscopic endoscopy showed that following resection, 97% of lesions were correctly anticipated to have sm2 + invasion. The specificity was relatively low at 50% showing that this

Table 8.2 The Kudo criteria for classifying pit patterns

Pit Type	Characteristics	Appearance using HMCC	Pit size (mm)
I	Normal round pits		0.07±0.02
II	Stellar or papillary		0.09±0.02
IIIs	Tubular/round pits Smaller than pit type I		0.03±0.01
IIIL	Tubular/large		0.22±0.09
IV	Sulcus/gyrus		0.93±0.32
V(a)	Irregular arrangement and sizes of IIIL, IIIs, IV type pit		N/A
V(n)	Non discemable		N/A

technique tended to over-stage lesions [58]. The concomitant use of high frequency ultrasound miniprobes may increase specificity and facilitate more accurate assessment of submucosal invasion, and thus select out those patients suitable for EMR. This involves the injection of a volume of saline into the submucosa to lift

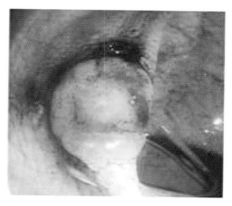 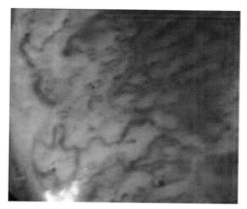

Figure 8.9   Type IIa + IIc lesion following indigo carmine dye spray. The lesion shows type Vn pits (absent pit staining) on HMCC, indicating submucosal invasion is likely. Histological examination confirmed early invasive adenocarcinoma.

the lesion and make it amenable to snare resection. Lesions that do not lift cleanly following submucosal injection may be invading the submucosal layer and are not suitable for EMR (non-lifting sign [59,60]).

In summary, endoscopic features which predict a high probability of submucosal invasion are: lesions which show depressed morphology and are greater than 15 mm in diameter; when the border of an elevated and depressed (0 – IIa + IIc) lesion is a smooth circle without indentations; when the non-lifting sign is present or there is an advanced pit pattern.

Other indications for ERUS in rectal cancer

In addition to pretreatment staging, ERUS may have a role in three other areas: identification of potential areas of invasive malignancy in apparently benign lesions; restaging of rectal cancer following neoadjuvant therapy; and in the detection of local recurrence.

ERUS and apparently benign lesions

It is recognized that between 30% and 40% of rectal villous adenomas contain areas of invasive carcinoma [61,62,63,64]. Even when adenomas with clinical features of malignancy (e.g., induration and ulceration) are excluded, approximately 10% of biopsy negative adenomas still contain foci of invasive carcinoma [61]. A recent meta-analysis [65] found that of 258 biopsy-negative rectal adenomas, 24% had focal carcinoma on histopathology. ERUS correctly identified cancer in 81% of these misdiagnosed lesions. They concluded that the use of ERUS for directed biopsy might be expected to decrease the need for additional surgery and other associated problems caused by misdiagnosis from 24% to 5%.

Role of ERUS in restaging rectal cancer following neoadjuvant therapy

Currently, ERUS has a limited role in assessing the response to neoadjuvant therapy. While it seems reasonable that restaging with ERUS could assess treatment response and help determine the most appropriate surgical approach, Vanagunas and colleagues [66] found ERUS to be inaccurate in this regard. This was because of its inability to differentiate tumor from radiation fibrosis. However, the use of ERUS-FNA was not evaluated and it may be here by way of its improved N-staging that ERUS-FNA has a role.

It remains to be seen if ERUS-FNA and other new imaging techniques such as FDG-PET [67] will assist in predicting the response to neoadjuvant therapy.

Early detection of locally recurrent rectal cancer

More than 90% of pelvic recurrence occurs within the first 36 months following surgery. Such patients have a poor prognosis with 80%–90% dying within 5 years of diagnosis [1,68,69,70]. To achieve cure by further surgery, it is necessary to detect recurrence early and ERUS has been found to be useful in this setting [70,71,72,73,74]. Both CT [75] and MRI [76] are effective methods for detecting recurrence but suffer from certain limitations. Whilst tumor diameter is less of a problem with multislice CT, low sensitivity for detecting lymph node metastases remains. Similarly, artifacts from metal clips and disruption of the normal anatomy by fibrosis or inflammation mimicking tumor recurrence can also be a factor. Tissue characterization by MRI is superior to CT but expense, limited availability and low patient compliance may prevent its routine use. Considerable enthusiasm exists over the use of FDG-PET [77,78,79] and immunoscintigraphy [80,81,82] in the detection of local recurrence, and initial reports suggest a future role.

By combining endoscopy (endoluminal tumor visualization) with ultrasound (extramural tumor visualization), ERUS is a valuable tool for detecting rectal cancer recurrence. Postsurgical or postradiation inflammatory changes can make the ultrasonic images difficult to evaluate but two prospective studies have demonstrated superior results with ERUS when compared with CT in detecting recurrence [83,84]. Furthermore, with the addition of FNA, Hunerbein *et al.* [85] found that ERUS-directed biopsy was significantly more accurate than CT or ERUS because of increased specificity.

It is important not to forget that a primary goal of follow-up in these patients is to detect recurrence as early as possible and thus facilitate curative re-intervention. A clear advantage of ERUS–FNA is its ability to detect and obtain tissue from very small pararectal recurrences [86] at an asymptomatic early stage, and longitudinal studies are awaited to ascertain whether or not identification of such patients will ultimately translate into improved long-term survival or cure. In the meantime, others argue that intensive follow-up is justified on the basis of improved quality and quantity of life offered by timely palliation of symptoms rather than last ditch procedures to obtain long-term survival in advanced disease [84].

Conclusion

Modern-day management of rectal cancer is often complex, reflecting the drive to minimize the chance of local recurrence and to improve long-term survival. Certainly, in locally advanced disease, there are clear benefits in the use of pre-operative radiotherapy with or without chemotherapy and MRI has been shown to be an accurate preoperative staging modality in such cases.

In early rectal cancer, numerous less invasive treatment options are now available but concerns exist as to whether local excision is adequate therapy for cure. Nonetheless, appropriate patient selection is of critical importance and ERUS is currently the most accurate modality available. Furthermore, high magnification chromoendoscopy may be complementary to ERUS by providing important endoscopic clues for further ultrasound imaging [87].

Finally, ERUS–FNA may have an impact on rectal cancer management through its ability to "problem solve" by targeting foci of potential disease and suspicious-looking lymph nodes.

REFERENCES

1. Abulafi, A. M. and Williams, N. S. Local recurrence of colorectal cancer: the problem, mechanisms, management and adjuvant therapy. *Br J Surg*, **81**:1 (1994), 7–19.
2. Improved survival with preoperative radiotherapy in resectable rectal cancer. Swedish Rectal Cancer Trial. *N Engl J Med*, **336**:14 (1997), 980–7.

3. Kapiteijn, E., *et al.* Preoperative radiotherapy combined with total mesorectal excision for resectable rectal cancer. *N Engl J Med*, **345**:9 (2001), 638–46.

4. Folkesson, J., *et al.* Swedish rectal cancer trial: long lasting benefits from radiotherapy on survival and local recurrence rate. *J Clin Oncol*, **23**:24 (2005), 5644–50.

5. Lahaye, M. J., *et al.* Imaging for predicting the risk factors – the circumferential resection margin and nodal disease – of local recurrence in rectal cancer: a meta-analysis. *Semin Ultrasound CT MR*, **26**:4 (2005), 259–68.

6. Kiesslich, R., *et al.* Perspectives of chromo and magnifying endoscopy: how, how much, when, and whom should we stain? *J Clin Gastroenterol*, **38**:1 (2004), 7–13.

7. Chiesura-Corona, M., *et al.* Rectal cancer: CT local staging with histopathologic correlation. *Abdom Imaging*, **26**:2 (2001), 134–8.

8. Angelelli, G., *et al.* Rectal carcinoma: CT staging with water as contrast medium. *Radiology*, **177**:2 (1990), 511–4.

9. Matsuoka, H., *et al.* A prospective comparison between multidetector-row computed tomography and magnetic resonance imaging in the preoperative evaluation of rectal carcinoma. *Am J Surg*, **185**:6 (2003), 556–9.

10. Taylor, A., *et al.* Preoperative staging of rectal cancer by MRI; results of a UK survey. *Clin Radiol*, **60**:5 (2005), 579–86.

11. Brown, G., *et al.* Rectal carcinoma: thin-section MR imaging for staging in 28 patients. *Radiology*, **211**:1 (1999), 215–22.

12. Beets-Tan, R. G., *et al.* Accuracy of magnetic resonance imaging in prediction of tumour-free resection margin in rectal cancer surgery. *Lancet*, **357**:9255 (2001), 497–504.

13. Heald, R. J., Husband, E. M., and Ryall, R. D. The mesorectum in rectal cancer surgery – the clue to pelvic recurrence? *Br J Surg*, **69**:10 (1982), 613–16.

14. Brown, G., *et al.* Preoperative assessment of prognostic factors in rectal cancer using high-resolution magnetic resonance imaging. *Br J Surg*, **90**:3 (2003), 355–64.

15. Wild, J. J. and Reid, J. M. Diagnostic use of ultrasound. *Br J Phys Med*, **19**:11 (1956), 248–57; passim.

16. Dragsted, J. and Gammelgaard, J. Endoluminal ultrasonic scanning in the evaluation of rectal cancer: a preliminary report of 13 cases. *Gastrointest Radiol*, **8**:4 (1983), 367–9.

17. Hildebrandt, U., *et al.* Significant improvement in clinical staging of rectal carcinoma with intrarectal ultrasound scanner. *J Exp Clin Cancer Res (suppl)*, **2**:53 (1983).

18. Rifkin, M. D. and Marks, G. J. Transrectal US as an adjunct in the diagnosis of rectal and extrarectal tumors. *Radiology*, **157**:2 (1985), 499–502.

19. Konishi, F., *et al.* Transrectal ultrasonography for the assessment of invasion of rectal carcinoma. *Dis Colon Rectum*, **28**:12 (1985), 889–94.

20. Beynon, J., *et al.* The endosonic appearances of normal colon and rectum. *Dis Colon Rectum*, **29**:12 (1986), 810–13.

21. Wiersema, M. J., *et al.* Endosonography-guided real-time fine-needle aspiration biopsy. *Gastrointest Endosc*, **40**:6 (1994), 700–7.

22. Vilmann, P., *et al.* Endoscopic ultrasonography with guided fine needle aspiration biopsy in pancreatic disease. *Gastrointest Endosc*, **38**:2 (1992), 172–3.

23. Chang, K. J., *et al.* Endoscopic ultrasound-guided fine-needle aspiration. *Gastrointest Endosc*, **40**:6 (1994), 694–9.

24. Milsom, J. W., *et al.* Preoperative biopsy of pararectal lymph nodes in rectal cancer using endoluminal ultrasonography. *Dis Colon Rectum*, **37**:4 (1994), 364–8.

25. Hawes, R. H. New staging techniques. Endoscopic ultrasound. *Cancer*, **71**:suppl. 12 (1993), 4207–13.

26. Glancy, D. G., Pullyblank, A. M., and Thomas, M. G. The role of colonoscopic endoanal ultrasound scanning (EUS) in selecting patients suitable for resection by transanal endoscopic microsurgery (TEM). *Colorectal Dis*, **7**:2 (2005), 148–50.

27. Savides, T. J. and Master, S. S. EUS in rectal cancer. *Gastrointest Endosc*, **56**:suppl. 4 (2002), S12–18.

28. Harewood, G. C. Assessment of publication bias in the reporting of EUS performance in staging rectal cancer. *Am J Gastroenterol*, **100**:4 (2005), 808–16.

29. Hulsmans, F. J., *et al.* Assessment of tumor infiltration depth in rectal cancer with transrectal sonography: caution is necessary. *Radiology*, **190**:3 (1994), 715–20.

30. Maier, A. G., *et al.* Peritumoral tissue reaction at transrectal US as a possible cause of overstaging in rectal cancer: histopathologic correlation. *Radiology*, **203**:3 (1997), 785–9.

31. Bhutani, M. S., Hawes, R. H., and Hoffman, B. J. A comparison of the accuracy of echo features during endoscopic ultrasound (EUS) and EUS-guided fine-needle aspiration for diagnosis of malignant lymph node invasion. *Gastrointest Endosc*, **45**:6 (1997), 474–9.

32. Pellise, M., *et al.* Detection of lymph node micrometastases by gene promoter hypermethylation in samples obtained by endosonography-guided fine-needle aspiration biopsy. *Clin Cancer Res*, **10**:13 (2004), 4444–9.

33. Harewood, G. C., *et al.* A prospective, blinded assessment of the impact of preoperative staging on the management of rectal cancer. *Gastroenterology*, **123**:1 (2002), 24–32.

34. Shami, V. M., Parmar, K. S., and Waxman, I. Clinical impact of endoscopic ultrasound and endoscopic ultrasound-guided fine-needle aspiration in the management of rectal carcinoma. *Dis Colon Rectum*, **47**:1 (2004), 59–65.

35. Brodsky, J. T., *et al.* Variables correlated with the risk of lymph node metastasis in early rectal cancer. *Cancer*, **69**:2 (1992), 322–6.

36. Zenni, G. C., *et al.* Characteristics of rectal carcinomas that predict the presence of lymph node metastases: implications for patient selection for local therapy. *J Surg Oncol*, **67**:2 (1998), 99–103.

37. Sitzler, P. J., *et al.* Lymph node involvement and tumor depth in rectal cancers: an analysis of 805 patients. *Dis Colon Rectum*, **40**:12 (1997), 1472–6.

38. Sengupta, S. and Tjandra, J. J. Local excision of rectal cancer: what is the evidence? *Dis Colon Rectum*, **44**:9 (2001), 1345–61.

39. Ogiwara, H., Nakamura, T., and Baba, S. Variables related to risk of recurrence in rectal cancer without lymph node metastasis. *Ann Surg Oncol*, **1**:2 (1994), 99–104.

40. Haggitt, R. C., *et al.* Prognostic factors in colorectal carcinomas arising in adenomas: implications for lesions removed by endoscopic polypectomy. *Gastroenterology*, **89**:2 (1985), 328–36.

41. Nivatvongs, S. Surgical management of early colorectal cancer. *World J Surg*, **24**:9 (2000), 1052–5.

42. Kudo, S. Endoscopic mucosal resection of flat and depressed types of early colorectal cancer. *Endoscopy*, **25**:7 (1993), 455–61.

43. Kikuchi, R., *et al.* Management of early invasive colorectal cancer. Risk of recurrence and clinical guidelines. *Dis Colon Rectum*, **38**:12 (1995), 1286–95.

44. Tanaka, S., *et al.* Endoscopic treatment of submucosal invasive colorectal carcinoma with special reference to risk factors for lymph node metastasis. *J Gastroenterol*, **30**:6 (1995), 710–7.

45. Akasu, T., *et al.* Endorectal ultrasonography and treatment of early stage rectal cancer. *World J Surg*, **24**:9 (2000), 1061–8.

46. Kudo, S., *et al.* Endoscopic diagnosis and treatment of early colorectal cancer. *World J Surg*, **21**:7 (1997), 694–701.

47. Harada, N., *et al.* Preoperative evaluation of submucosal invasive colorectal cancer using a 15-MHz ultrasound miniprobe. *Endoscopy*, **33**:3 (2001), 237–40.

48. Muto, T., *et al.* Small "flat adenoma" of the large bowel with special reference to its clinico-pathologic features. *Dis Colon Rectum*, **28**:11 (1985), 847–51.

49. Rembacken, B. J., *et al.* Flat and depressed colonic neoplasms: a prospective study of 1000 colonoscopies in the UK. *Lancet*, **355**:9211 (2000), 1211–14.

50. Saitoh, Y., *et al.* Prevalence and distinctive biologic features of flat colorectal adenomas in a North American population. *Gastroenterology*, **120**:7 (2001), 1657–65.

51. Tsuda, S., *et al.* Flat and depressed colorectal tumours in a southern Swedish population: a prospective chromoendoscopic and histopathological study. *Gut*, **51**:4 (2002), 550–5.

52. Hurlstone, D. P., *et al.* A prospective clinicopathological and endoscopic evaluation of flat and depressed colorectal lesions in the United Kingdom. *Am J Gastroenterol*, **98**:11 (2003), 2543–9.

53. Suzuki, N., Talbot, I. C., and Saunders, B. P. The prevalence of small, flat colorectal cancers in a western population. *Colorectal Dis*, **6**:1 (2004), 15–20.

54. General rules for clinical and pathological studies on cancer of the colon, rectum and anus. Part I. Clinical classification. Japanese Research Society for Cancer of the Colon and Rectum. *Jpn J Surg*, **13**:6 (1983), 557–73.

55. Update on the paris classification of superficial neoplastic lesions in the digestive tract. *Endoscopy*, **37**:6 (2005), 570–8.

56. The Paris endoscopic classification of superficial neoplastic lesions: esophagus, stomach, and colon: November 30 to December 1, 2002. *Gastrointest Endosc*, **58**:suppl. 6 (2003), S3–43.

57. Kudo, S., *et al.* Pit pattern in colorectal neoplasia: endoscopic magnifying view. *Endoscopy*, **33**:4 (2001), 367–73.

58. Hurlstone, D. P., *et al.* Endoscopic morphological anticipation of submucosal invasion in flat and depressed colorectal lesions: clinical implications and subtype analysis of the kudo type V pit pattern using high-magnification-chromoscopic colonoscopy. *Colorectal Dis*, **6**:5 (2004), 369–75.

59. Uno, Y. and Munakata, A. The non-lifting sign of invasive colon cancer. *Gastrointest Endosc*, **40**:4 (1994), 485–9.

60. Kato, H., *et al.* Lifting of lesions during endoscopic mucosal resection (EMR) of early colorectal cancer: implications for the assessment of resectability. *Endoscopy*, **33**:7 (2001), 568–73.

61. Nivatvongs, S., *et al.* Villous adenomas of the rectum: the accuracy of clinical assessment. *Surgery*, **87**:5 (1980), 549–51.

62. Galandiuk, S., *et al.* Villous and tubulovillous adenomas of the colon and rectum. A retrospective review, 1964–1985. *Am J Surg*, **153**:1 (1987), 41–7.

63. Taylor, E. W., *et al.* Limitations of biopsy in preoperative assessment of villous papilloma. *Dis Colon Rectum*, **24**:4 (1981), 259–62.

64. Christiansen, J., Kirkegaard, P., and Ibsen, J. Prognosis after treatment of villous adenomas of the colon and rectum. *Ann Surg*, **189**:4 (1979), 404–8.

65. Worrell, S., *et al.* Endorectal ultrasound detection of focal carcinoma within rectal adenomas. *Am J Surg*, **187**:5 (2004), 625–9, discussion 629.

66. Vanagunas, A., Lin, D. E., and Stryker, S. J. Accuracy of endoscopic ultrasound for restaging rectal cancer following neoadjuvant chemoradiation therapy [see comment]. *Am J Gastroenterol*, **99**:1 (2004), 109–12.

67. Amthauer, H., *et al.* Response prediction by FDG-PET after neoadjuvant radiochemotherapy and combined regional hyperthermia of rectal cancer: correlation with endorectal ultrasound and histopathology. *Eur J Nucl Med Mol Imaging*, **31**:6 (2004), 811–19.

68. Schiessel, R., Wunderlich, M., and Herbst, F. Local recurrence of colorectal cancer: effect of early detection and aggressive surgery. *Br J Surg*, **73**:5 (1986), 342–4.

69. Wanebo, H. J., *et al.* Pelvic resection of recurrent rectal cancer. *Ann Surg*, **220**:4 (1994), 586–95, discussion 595–7.

70. Romano, G., *et al.* Impact of computed tomography vs. intrarectal ultrasound on the diagnosis, resectability, and prognosis of locally recurrent rectal cancer. *Dis Colon Rectum*, **36**:3 (1993), 261–5.

71. Beynon, J., *et al.* The detection and evaluation of locally recurrent rectal cancer with rectal endosonography. *Dis Colon Rectum*, **32**:6 (1989), 509–17.

72. Mascagni, D., *et al.* Endoluminal ultrasound for early detection of local recurrence of rectal cancer. *Br J Surg*, **76**:11 (1989), 1176–80.

73. Scialpi, M., *et al.* Rectal carcinoma: preoperative staging and detection of postoperative local recurrence with transrectal and transvaginal ultrasound. *Abdom Imaging*, **18**:4 (1993), 381–9.

74. Milsom, J. W., *et al.* The expanding utility of endoluminal ultrasonography in the management of rectal cancer. *Surgery*, **112**:4 (1992), 832–40, discussion 840–1.

75. Tanaka, J., *et al.* Usefulness of early-phase helical CT for detecting recurrent rectal cancer. *Radiat Med*, **21**:3 (2003), 103–7.

76. Torricelli, P., *et al.* Gadolinium-enhanced MRI with dynamic evaluation in diagnosing the local recurrence of rectal cancer. *Abdom Imaging*, **28**:1 (2003), 19–27.

77. Moore, H. G., *et al.* A case-controlled study of 18-fluorodeoxyglucose positron emission tomography in the detection of pelvic recurrence in previously irradiated rectal cancer patients. *J Am Coll Surg*, **197**:1 (2003), 22–8.

78. Fukunaga, H., *et al.* Fusion image of positron emission tomography and computed tomography for the diagnosis of local recurrence of rectal cancer. *Ann Surg Oncol*, **12**:7 (2005), 561–9.

79. Arulampalam, T. H., *et al.* Positron emission tomography and colorectal cancer. *Br J Surg*, **88**:2 (2001), 176–89.

80. Jarv, V., *et al.* Added value of CEA scintigraphy in the detection of recurrence of rectal carcinoma. *Acta Radiol*, **41**:6 (2000), 629–33.

81. Sirisriro, R., *et al.* Detection of colorectal carcinoma by anti-CEA monoclonal antibody (IOR-CEA1) labeled with 99mTc scintigraphy. *Hepatogastroenterology*, **47**:32 (2000), 405–13.

82. Ghesani, M., Belgraier, A., and Hasni, S. Carcinoembryonic antigen (CEA) scan in the diagnosis of recurrent colorectal carcinoma in a patient with increasing CEA levels and inconclusive computed tomographic findings. *Clin Nucl Med*, **28**:7 (2003), 608–9.

83. Novell, F., *et al.* Endorectal ultrasonography in the follow-up of rectal cancer. Is it a better way to detect early local recurrence? *Int J Colorectal Dis*, **12**:2 (1997), 78–81.

84. Rotondano, G., *et al.* Early detection of locally recurrent rectal cancer by endosonography. *Br J Radiol*, **70**:834 (1997), 567–71.

85. Hunerbein, M., *et al.* The role of transrectal ultrasound-guided biopsy in the postoperative follow-up of patients with rectal cancer. *Surgery*, **129**:2 (2001), 164–9.

86. Lohnert, M. S., Doniec, J. M., and Henne-Bruns, D. Effectiveness of endoluminal sonography in the identification of occult local rectal cancer recurrences. *Dis Colon Rectum*, **43**:4 (2000), 483–91.

87. Hurlstone, D. P., *et al.* High-magnification-chromoscopic-colonoscopy or high-frequency 20 MHz mini-probe endoscopic ultrasound staging for early colorectal neoplasia: a comparative prospective analysis. *Gut*, **54**:11 (2005), 1585–9.

9

CT staging

Sarah Burton and Gina Brown

Abstract

The role of CT in local staging of colorectal cancer is currently limited as the sensitivity for local invasion is reported as only 48%–55%. Soft tissue extending into the perirectal/colic fat is non-specific but the demonstration of T4 invasion in colorectal cancer may alter the surgical approach. In colon cancer, the preoperative assessment of T and N stage does not currently affect the preoperative treatment plan but this may change in the future. Nevertheless, CT is recommended in the preoperative assessment of colorectal tumors since it is useful for detection of complications related to the primary tumor (such as obstruction, perforation, and abscess formation) and will reliably detect metastatic disease.

CT in local staging of colorectal cancer

In patients with a known diagnosis of colon cancer, the use of preoperative staging using CT has been controversial. However, with improved CT techniques and the increasing use of preoperative therapy (e.g., in patients with potentially resectable synchronous disease), CT increasingly plays an important role in preoperative management. The optimal technique for imaging of the colon has already been described in detail in Chapter 3. For assessing local infiltration of the primary tumor, intravenous contrast enhancement is essential; oral contrast (usually 1000–1500 ml of oral water or air insufflation if colonography is being used) abdominal assessment should include thorax and liver to identify potentially resectable metastatic disease.

When spiral or multidetector CT is used, a 1.5–5-mm collimation is performed with scans acquired through the abdomen during the hepatic venous phase of liver enhancement, 50–60 seconds after the start of contrast material injection, to optimize detection of hepatic metastases.

T-staging

Since CT has not previously been shown to accurately stratify patients for local tumor spread, its present use is essentially limited to the assessment of distant metastases and evaluation of complications such as obstruction or perforation [1]. Indeed, several studies have questioned the routine use of preoperative CT scanning for staging colon cancers owing to its limited role in altering surgical management [2,3]. Accurate staging using CT is challenging since there is often insufficient contrast resolution to adequately depict spread external to the muscularis propria [4,5,6]. Invasion into adjacent structures (T4 disease) relies on the loss of fat planes between tumor and the adjacent organ (Figure 9.1), and overstaging of T4 disease may occur because of inflammation or cachexia-related loss of intra-abdominal or pelvic fat [7]. Freeny *et al.* demonstrated only 48% accuracy for predicting Dukes' classification in 80 patients with 9% overstaged and 44%

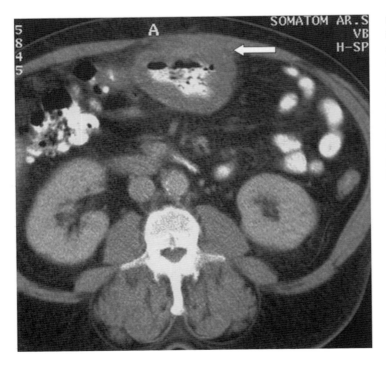

Figure 9.1 CT image in a male patient showing a transverse colon tumor as annular low-density thickening of the transverse colon. There is loss of the fat plane between the tumor and the anterior abdominal wall indicating T4 infiltration.

Table 9.1 CT image interpretation

Prognostic feature	Stage	CT criteria
T-stage	T1	Intraluminal projection of a colonic lesion without any visible distortion of the bowel wall layers
	T2	Asymmetrical thickening > 3 mm extending intraluminally without penetration of the presumed site of muscularis propria
	T3	Peritumoral stranding
		Smooth extension of a discrete mass beyond the expected site of muscularis propria
		Peritumoral nodularity
	T4	Irregular elevation of the outer layer (peritoneum) of the bowel wall
		Irregular advancing edge of tumor penetrating adjacent organs
		Loss of well-defined plane between peritoneum and adjacent structures
Nodal status	N0	No lymph nodes greater than 1 cm and no abnormal clustering
	N1	1–3 lymph nodes > 1 cm or abnormal clustering of 3 or more normal sized lymph nodes
	N2	More than 3 lymph nodes >1 cm
EMVI	Absent	No tumor extension visible within colic vessels
	Present	Nodularity of colic vessels indicating invasion by tumor
RSM	Clear	≥ 1 mm clearance from posterior fascia
	Involved	Blurring of the posterior fascia indicating tumor extending to the posterior resection margin

understaged [8]. Nevertheless, most patients will undergo a preoperative CT examination of the thorax, abdomen, and pelvis to assess metastatic disease; and with a clear understanding of the anatomical and pathological prognostic considerations in colon cancer, potentially useful staging information can be obtained (Table 9.1). The main criterion for identification of tumor is focal thickening of the colonic wall (Figure 9.2) [9,10,11]. Extension into pericolic tissues is indicated by irregularity of the border of the colonic wall and strands of soft tissue extending into perirectal fat (Figure 9.3) [7,12]. If a prognostic score is used to simplify stage into good or bad depending on absence of T4 and N2 (good) or presence of either T4 or N2 (bad),

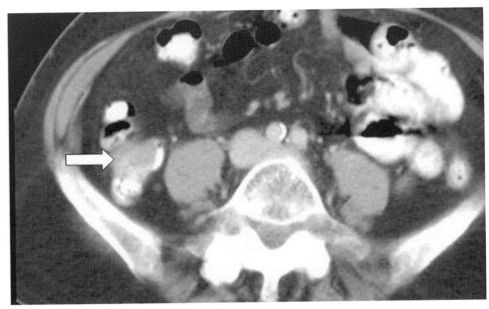

Figure 9.2   CT image of cecal tumor in a female patient. The primary tumor can be demonstrated as focal low-density thickening arising from the colonic wall (arrow).

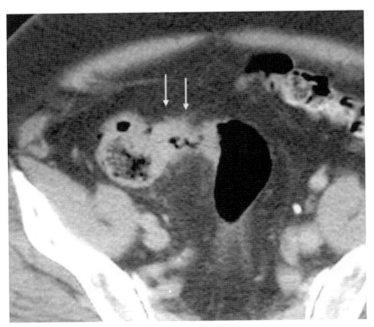

Figure 9.3   CT image of a sigmoid/descending colon tumor in a male patient. There is focal thickening and enhancement representing primary tumor and in addition nodular stranding of soft tissue density is demonstrated in the pericolonic fat (arrows) indicating infiltration through and beyond the colonic wall.

better agreement with histopathology can be achieved and indicate potential for using CT scanning as a tool for preoperatively identifying patients with poor prognosis who may benefit from neoadjuvant therapies [13].

Anatomical considerations in staging

The cecum, ascending colon, and descending colon are covered anteriorly by visceral peritoneum which extends medially onto the rudimentary mesocolon and laterally onto the abdominal wall as parietal peritoneum. Therefore, approximately 50% of the posterior circumference at these sites of the colon is free of peritoneum. This has been described as the "bare area" or retroperitoneal surgical margin (RSM) and is the plane of dissection during surgical resection. Involvement of this area by tumor would indicate T3 disease with a positive margin rather than peritoneal involvement (T4 disease). In contrast, the transverse and sigmoid colon are completely invested in peritoneum and are suspended on their respective mesenteries. Therefore, the RSM in these regions is minimal and will only occur at the root of the mesentery where the colonic vessels will be ligated (Figure 9.4).

Previous studies have described the criteria for predicting local extension of tumor beyond muscularis propria as a discrete mass or focal thickening of the bowel wall [14]. The usual bowel wall thickness on CT is 3 mm with 6 mm being considered abnormal [15]. Asymmetrical bowel wall thickening with or without an irregular surface is likely to be tumor (Figure 9.5). A smooth outer margin has been reported to predict tumor within the bowel wall as well as an absence of stranding in the pericolic fat [15] (Figure 9.6). Nodularity or peritumoral stranding are useful indications of T3 disease. In contrast to T3 rectal tumors whereof penetration beyond muscularis propria can be clearly seen within the mesorectal fat pad, the anatomy of the colon and the lack of an anatomically well-defined mesocolon make this prognostic feature much more difficult to observe.

T4 disease or evidence of peritoneal involvement, with or without penetration of adjacent organs has been shown to be a poor prognostic indicator in colon cancer [16]. Peritoneal involvement without invasion of adjacent organs can be difficult to predict as the serosa is a particularly thin layer of the bowel wall. Previous studies have not described T staging of tumors in the context of peritoneal anatomy but instead have limited assessment of T4 staging as invasion into adjacent organs shown by loss of fat planes [15]. Using different criteria (Table 9.1) and with knowledge of peritonealized surfaces of the colon, accuracies of 70%–85% can be achieved through an understanding of peritonealized vs.

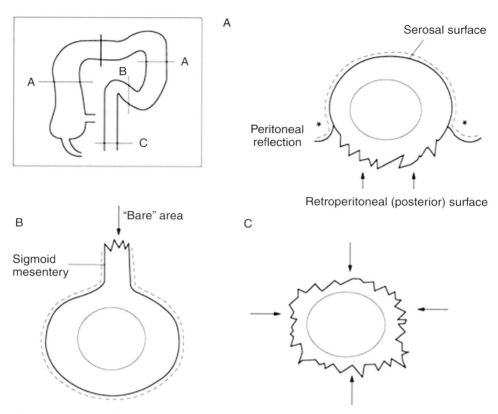

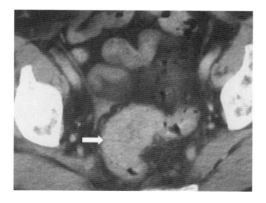

Figure 9.4   Diagram illustrating the serosal surfaces vs. retroperitoneal surgical margins according to location within the colon and rectum. A = ascending or descending colon; B = sigmoid colon and transverse colon; C = rectum.

Figure 9.5   CT image of sigmoid tumor showing focal thickening and enhancement (arrow), but no nodular enhancement beyond the contour of the bowel wall indicating T2 or minimal T3 disease.

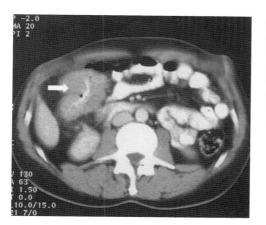

Figure 9.6 CT image of a bulky cecal tumor with circumferential thickening and low attenuation of the cecal wall. The contour of the bowel wall does not appear obviously disrupted indicating T2 or minimal T3 disease. Histology of the final specimen showed T3 disease illustrating the difficulty in distinguishing early T3 and T2 tumors using CT.

non-peritonealized colonic surfaces (Figure 9.7). Extramural vascular invasion is a reported poor prognostic factor in colon cancer resulting in reduced overall and disease-free survival [17]. It has previously been identified using MRI in rectal cancer and is described as serpiginous extension of tumor within a vascular structure [18]. We have recently reported the visualization of extramural vascular invasion (EMVI) on CT [19]. By using similar criteria as described above for MR imaging in rectal cancer, it is possible to identify this feature on CT. Nodularity of the vessel involved appears to be the most consistent feature of EMVI on CT (Figure 9.8).

In rectal cancer, positive circumferential margins have been shown to be a predictor for local recurrence and systemic failure [20,21,22,23]. The non-peritonealized "bare" area or retroperitoneal resection margin (RSM) has recently been described for right-sided colonic tumors with the incidence of positive margins at 7% [24] coinciding with other reported series of colonic local recurrences of 6%–10% [25,26]. A similar "bare" area can also be defined for the descending colon.

The frequency of RSM involvement in colon cancers [24] is substantially less than CRM involvement in rectal cancers [20] but contributes to local recurrence in these patients. Better tumor-free resection margins in colon cancer can be attributed to the relative ease of achieving a clear resection during colonic resection compared with the rather limited clearance potential in the pelvis with rectal cancers. Larger studies are therefore needed to determine whether preoperative RSM status is a useful predictor of poor prognosis in colon cancers. It is defined on CT as tumor lying within 1 mm of the retroperitoneal fascia (Figures 9.9 and 9.10).

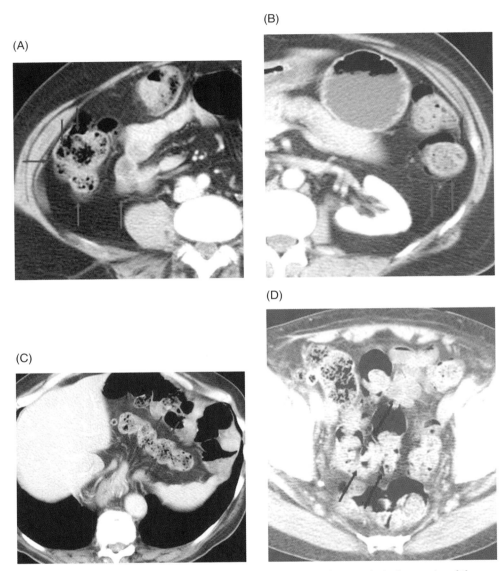

Figure 9.7 CT demonstration of the retroperitoneal surgical resection margin (red arrows) and the peritoneum (green arrows) in (A) the ascending colon and (B) the descending colon Figure 1 CT demonstration of complete investment of (C) transverse colon and (D) sigmoid colon by peritoneum (green arrows).

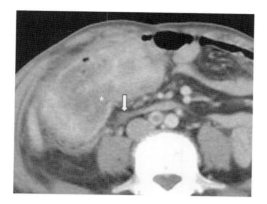

Figure 9.8   Axial CT scan showing an ascending colon tumor (*). The ileocolic vessel is demonstrated and this is irregular and somewhat nodular contour (arrow). This appearance has been shown to correspond to venous invasion by tumor.

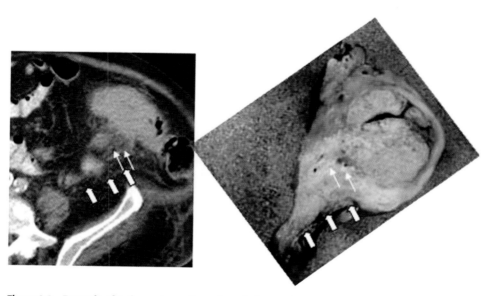

Figure 9.9   Example of a clear retroperitoneal surgical resection margin. Here, a descending colon tumor is demonstrated (arrow) and infiltration of tumor is demonstrated along the mesenteric border, however, this does not extend to the retroperitoneal surgical resection plane (wide arrows) and this is confirmed on the subsequent histopathology section.

It is also of value to note the presence or absence of a complication related to the primary tumor. These include

- Intestinal obstruction
- Local tumor perforation/fistula formation
- Pericolic abscess

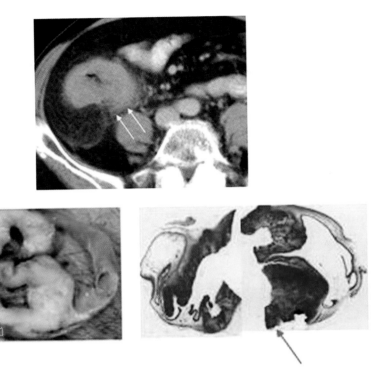

Figure 9.10 Example of tumor extending to the retroperitoneal surgical resection margin. A cecal tumor is demonstrated with posterior infiltration of tumor, which extends to the posterior fascia. Surgical resection resulted in a positive surgical margin (arrows).

- Intussusception
- Acute appendicitis.

Intestinal obstruction is the most common complication of carcinoma of the colon and has an unfavorable effect upon prognosis. Such patients often present with more advanced disease and in such circumstances, primary surgery is seldom curative [27]. Penetration of the wall of the colon by carcinoma is sometimes associated with the development of a pericolic abscess which can then lead to local recurrence (Figure 9.11). Other complications include intussusception of the colon (Figure 9.12), which in adults is more often because of carcinoma than a benign cause [28] and on occasion, an acute appendicitis may be a presenting feature owing to tumor growth in the right colon producing back pressure and appendiceal obstruction [29]. Local tumor perforation (Figure 9.13) through the peritoneal membrane is common and also indicates an unfavorable prognosis; this is not only because of associated peritonitis, but also because of the risk of dissemination

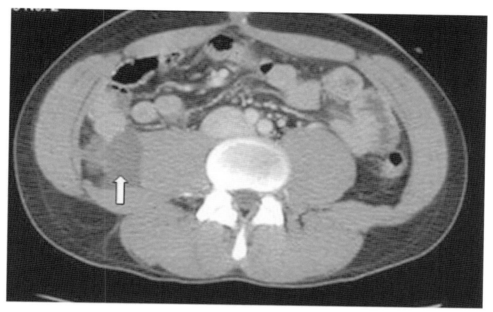

Figure 9.11   CT scan showing mucinous recurrence (arrow) in a patient with previously perforated cecal carcinoma.

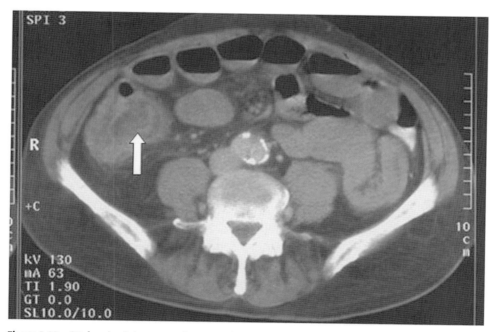

Figure 9.12   CT showing intussuscepting ascending colon tumor (arrow).

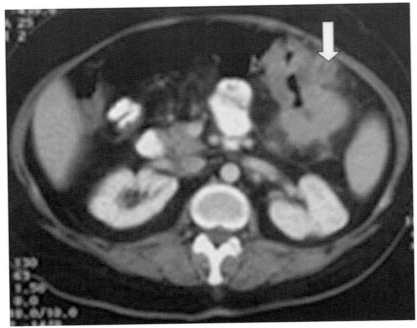

Figure 9.13   CT scan showing transverse colon tumor. Anteriorly, the transverse colon is covered by serosa, so tumor extension beyond the contour anteriorly is highly likely to represent T4 peritoneal perforation as is shown in this example (arrow).

of malignant cells within the abdomen resulting in transcoelomic spread and peritoneal involvement (Figure 9.14) [16]. Tumor cells may be present in peritoneal washings in up to 42% of patients [30]. Transcoelomic metastases favor certain sites, such as to the lower right small bowel mesentery (superior and inferior ileocolic recesses), the intersigmoid recess, and the rectovesical or rectouterine pouch (pouch of Douglas) [31,32].

N-staging

Knowledge of the expected site of nodes will assist in their CT identification. The lymphatic vessels run along the course of the vessels arcading within the mesocolon and beneath the peritoneum of the posterior abdominal wall. There are three main groups of lymph nodes. The first group are the paracolic lymph nodes which lie in the peritoneum close to the colon. The second group lie along the main vessels supplying blood to the colon. The third group are the para-aortic nodes which cluster around the root of the SMA and IMA and are classified as distant

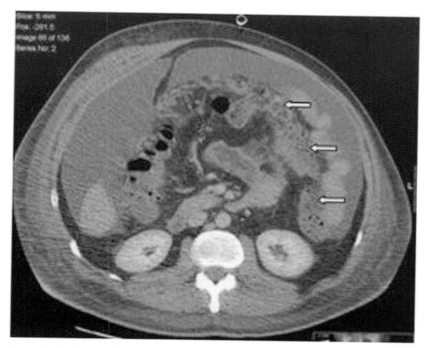

Figure 9.14   CT scan showing an example of extensive peritoneal disease. There are widespread plaques of peritoneal infiltration (arrows).

metastases. Whilst rectal lymph nodes are confined within a well-defined mesor-ectal envelope, colonic lymph nodes spread along the much broader mesentery. Nodes over 1 cm are usually predicted as positive on CT and although this criterion is specific, it has a very poor sensitivity [33], and this inaccuracy relates to reliance on size criteria which results in both overstaging of enlarged nodes and under-staging of normal-sized nodes (Figure 9.15). The large comparative study reported by the RDOG [10] found a sensitivity for detecting lymph node metastases in 322 patients to be 38% for rectal cancer and 56% for colon cancer; the overall accuracy in all patients studied was only 62%. Previous studies have successfully demon-strated nodal metastases using CT by following the lymph drainage along the vascular supply [34,35]. It is unlikely that CT imaging will be able to assess lymph node status sufficiently accurately to influence outcomes as no imaging technique will consistently identify small 2–3 mm foci of metastatic disease within normal-sized lymph nodes.

T4 stage, N2 stage, EMVI positivity, and emergency presentation are indepen-dent predictors of poor prognosis. Emergency presentations cannot be predicted

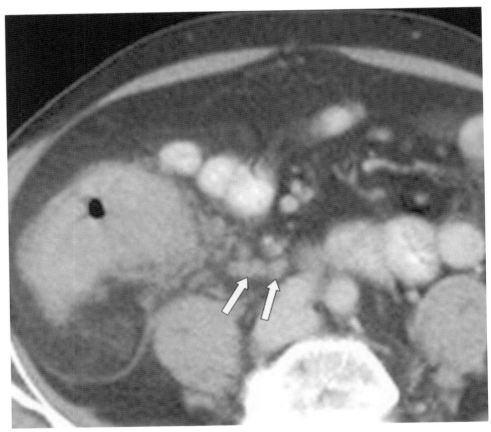

Figure 9.15   CT scan showing an example of enlarged and enhancing lymph nodes along the ileocolic vessels (arrows). Prediction of nodal status is insufficiently accurate using these criteria.

preoperatively and are also of prognostic significance. However, if the implementation of a preoperative strategy similar to that of rectal cancer can be shown to be effective in colon cancer, then emergency surgical management of obstructed tumors may alter; defunctioning ileostomy/colostomy or stenting rather than primary resection of the tumor may become appropriate to allow adequate staging and downsizing of advanced tumors. In the non-emergency situation, poor prognostic features such as locally extensive T3 and T4 disease and presence of EMVI may be predicted preoperatively by appropriate imaging. In recent years, the paradigm for treatment of patients with solid tumors has shifted from postoperative adjuvant therapy to neoadjuvant therapy prior to definitive surgery. In patients with colorectal cancer, the potential benefits are greatest for those at high risk of systemic failure, therefore preoperative identification of these features and stratification of patients into prognostic groups will be important in future management. Improvements in CT may enable more accurate identification of poor prognostic features known to reduce disease-free and overall survival in colon cancers.

REFERENCES

1. Horton, K. M., Abrams, R. A., and Fishman, E. K. Spiral CT of colon cancer: imaging features and role in management. *Radiographics*, **20**:2 (2000), 419–30.

2. McAndrew, M. R. and Saba, A. K. Efficacy of routine preoperative computed tomography scans in colon cancer. *Am Surg*, **65**:3 (1999), 205–8.

3. Barton, J. B., Langdale, L. A., Cummins, J. S., *et al.* The utility of routine preoperative computed tomography scanning in the management of veterans with colon cancer. *Am J Surg*, **183**:5 (2002), 499–503.

4. Butch, R. J., Stark, D. D., Wittenberg, J., *et al.* Staging rectal cancer by MR and CT. *AJR Am J Roentgenol*, **146**:6 (1986), 1155–60.

5. Rifkin, M. D. and Wechsler, R. J. A comparison of computed tomography and endorectal ultrasound in staging rectal cancer. *Int J Colorectal Dis*, **1**:4 (1986), 219–23.

6. Holdsworth, P. J., Johnston, D., Chalmers, A. G., *et al.* Endoluminal ultrasound and computed tomography in the staging of rectal cancer. *Br J Surg*, **75**:10 (1988), 1019–22.

7. Thoeni, R. F. CT evaluation of carcinomas of the colon and rectum. *Radiol Clin North Am*, **27**:4 (1989), 731–41.

8. Freeny, P. C., Marks, W. M., Ryan, J. A., and Bolen, J. W. Colorectal carcinoma evaluation with CT: preoperative staging and detection of postoperative recurrence. *Radiology*, **158**:2 (1986), 347–53.

9. Mehta, S., Johnson, R. J., and Schofield, P. F. Staging of colorectal cancer. *Clin Radiol*, **49**:8 (1994), 515–23.

10. Zerhouni, E. A., Rutter, C., Hamilton, S. R., *et al.* CT and MR imaging in the staging of colorectal carcinoma: report of the Radiology Diagnostic Oncology Group II. *Radiology*, **200**:2 (1996), 443–51.

11. Kim, N. K., Kim, M. J., Yun, S. H., Sohn, S. K., and Min, J. S. Comparative study of transrectal ultrasonography, pelvic computerized tomography, and magnetic resonance imaging in pre-operative staging of rectal cancer. *Dis Colon Rectum*, **42**:6 (1999), 770–5.

12. Thoeni, R. F., Moss, A. A., Schnyder, P., and Margulis, A. R. Detection and staging of primary rectal and rectosigmoid cancer by computed tomography. *Radiology*, **141**:1 (1981), 135–8.

13. Smith, N. J., Bees, N. Predicting prognosis in colon cancer: validation of a new pre-operative CT staging classification and implications for clinical trials. *Colorectal Dis*, **8**:suppl. 2 (2006), 18.

14. Thoeni, R. F. Colorectal cancer: cross-sectional imaging for staging of primary tumor and detection of local recurrence. *AJR Am J Roentgenol*, **156**:5 (1991), 909–15.

15. Thoeni, R. F. Colorectal cancer. Radiologic staging. *Radiol Clin North Am*, **35**:2 (1997), 457–85.

16. Shepherd, N. A., Baxter, K. J., and Love, S. B. The prognostic importance of peritoneal involvement in colonic cancer: a prospective evaluation. *Gastroenterology*, **112**:4 (1997), 1096–102.

17. Chapuis, P. H., Dent, O. F., Bokey, E. L., Newland, R. C., and Sinclair, G., *et al.* Adverse histopathological findings as a guide to patient management after curative resection of node-positive colonic cancer. *Br J Surg*, **91**:3 (2004), 349–54.

18. Chau, I., Allen, M., Cummingham, D., *et al.* Neoadjuvant systemic fluorouracil and mitomycin C prior to synchronous chemoradiation is an effective strategy in locally advanced rectal cancer. *Br J Cancer*, **88**:7 (2003), 1017–24.

19. Burton, S., Brown, G., Bees, N., *et al.* Accuracy of MRI prediction of poor prognostic features in colonic cancer. *Colorectal Dis*, **8**:suppl. 2 (2006).

20. Adam, I. J., Mohamdee, M. O., Martin, I. G., *et al.* Role of circumferential margin involvement in the local recurrence of rectal cancer. *Lancet*, **344**:8924 (1994), 707–11.

21. Hall, N. R., Finan, P. J., al-Jaberi, T., *et al.* Circumferential margin involvement after mesorectal excision of rectal cancer with curative intent. Predictor of survival but not local recurrence? *Dis Colon Rectum*, **41**:8 (1998), 979–83.

22. Birbeck, K. F., Macklin, C. P., Tiffin, N. J., *et al.* Rates of circumferential resection margin involvement vary between surgeons and predict outcomes in rectal cancer surgery. *Ann Surg*, **235**:4 (2002), 449–57.

23. Wibe, A., Rendedal, P. R., Svensson, E., *et al.* Prognostic significance of the circumferential resection margin following total mesorectal excision for rectal cancer. *Br J Surg*, **89**:3 (2002), 327–34.

24. Bateman, A. C., Carr, N. J., and Warren, B. F. The retroperitoneal surface in distal caecal and proximal ascending colon carcinoma: the Cinderella surgical margin? *J Clin Pathol*, **58**:4 (2005), 426–8.

25. Willett, C., Tepper, J. E., Cohen, A., *et al.* Local failure following curative resection of colonic adenocarcinoma. *Int J Radiat Oncol Biol Phys*, **10**:5 (1984), 645–51.

26. Carraro, P. G., Segala, M., Cesana, B. M., and Tiberio, G. Obstructing colonic cancer: failure and survival patterns over a ten-year follow-up after one-stage curative surgery. *Dis Colon Rectum*, **44**:2 (2001), 243–50.

27. Fielding, L. P., Phillips, R. K., Fry, J. S., and Hittinger, R. Prediction of outcome after curative resection for large bowel cancer. *Lancet*, **2**:8512 (1986), 904–7.

28. Aston, S. J. and Machlfeder, H. I. Intussusception in the adult. *Am Surg*, **41**:9 (1975), 576–80.

29. Arnbjornsson, E. Acute appendicitis as a sign of a colorectal carcinoma. *J Surg Oncol*, **20**:1 (1982), 17–20.

30. Wong, L. S., Morris, A. G., and Fraser, I. A. The exfoliation of free malignant cells in the peritoneal cavity during resection of colorectal cancer. *Surg Oncol*, 5 (1996), 115–21.

31. DeMeo, J. H., Fulcher, A. S., and Austin, R. F. Anatomic CT demonstration of the peritoneal spaces, ligaments and mesenteries: normal and pathologic processes. *Radiographics*, 15 (1995), 755–70.

32. Coakley, F. V. and Hricak, H. Imaging of peritoneal and mesenteric disease: key concepts for the clinical radiologist. *Clin Radiol*, **54**:9 (1999), 563–74.

33. Acunas, B., Rozanes, I., Acunas, G., Celik, L., Sayi, I., and Gokemen, E. Preoperative CT staging of colon carcinoma (excluding the recto-sigmoid region). *Eur J Radiol*, **11**:2 (1990), 150–3.

34. Granfield, C. A., Charnsangavej, C., and Dubrow, R. A., *et al*. Regional lymph node metastases in carcinoma of the left side of the colon and rectum: CT demonstration. *AJR Am J Roentgenol*, **159**:4 (1992), 757–61.

35. McDaniel, K. P., Charnsangavej, C., DuBrow, R. A., Varma, D. G., Granfield, C. A., and Curley, S. A., *et al*. Pathways of nodal metastasis in carcinomas of the cecum, ascending colon, and transverse colon: CT demonstration. *AJR Am J Roentgenol* **161**:1 (1993), 61–4.

10

MRI staging

Sarah Burton and Gina Brown

Abstract

High-resolution MR images show a high degree of resemblance to pathology sections, and with careful interpretation of the images, further important prognostic information that supplements the T and N staging can be obtained thus providing a method of selecting the intensity of preoperative therapy. Hitherto, these variables would only have been detected on the final operative specimen thus missing the opportunity to potentially downstage poor prognosis tumors and influence outcome. The success of preoperative therapy over postoperative treatments means that a technique identifying these factors preoperatively is of potential benefit in modifying the intensity of preoperative therapy according to prognosis. Increasingly, clinical trials are incorporating MR assessment of prognostic factors prior to therapy to enable objective comparison of treatment modalities and outcomes that are targeted to preoperative prognostic subgroups. By comparing pretreatment MR staging with posttherapy histology assessment, a quantifiable assessment of the efficacy of particular treatment protocols can be achieved.

The role of imaging in surgical planning

Colorectal cancer surgery is undertaken according to the following principles:

- Removal of colon or rectum together with the draining lymph nodes. The former by removal of its attached mesentery containing nodes (Figure 10.1), the latter achieved through en bloc removal of the mesorectum (Figure 10.2).
- Anal sphincter preservation unless tumor encroached upon the anal sphincter complex.
- Autonomic nerve preservation – this is particularly critical in rectal cancer surgery. The preoperative assessment of tumor prior to surgery and detailed discussion of the findings optimizes outcomes [1].

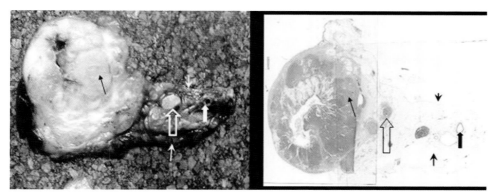

Figure 10.1   Cross-cut section and histology large section preparation (H & E stained) demonstrating a typical appearance of colon resection specimen. Cross-cut section of bowel wall containing tumor (black arrow) is demonstrated as well as the segment of the colonic mesentery (white arrow), which contains draining lymph nodes (open arrow) and vessels (block arrow).

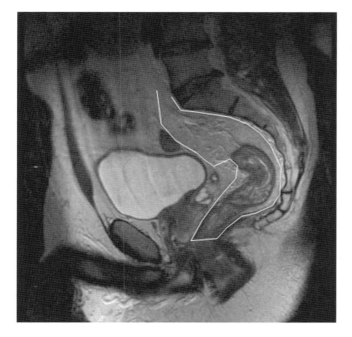

Figure 10.2   Sagittal MRI showing the planes of excision used in TME surgery.

The ability to clear the tumor in a curative procedure depends on the demonstration that:

● The tumor is clear of adjacent structures; namely, the prostate, seminal vesicles, bladder, and pelvic sidewalls in the case of sigmoid and rectal cancers (Figure 10.3) and the duodenum, other loops of small bowel and superior mesenteric vessels in the case of colonic tumors (Figure 10.4).

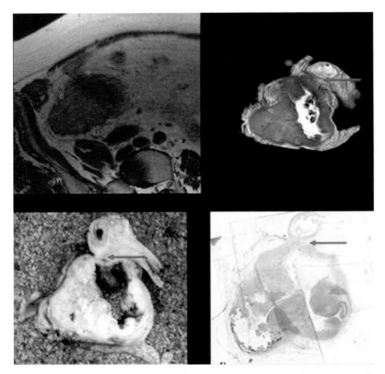

Figure 10.3   Axial MRI showing a polypoidal colonic tumor with anterior infiltration (arrow) and invasion towards a loop of small bowel indicating T4 disease (arrows). Corresponding histopathology and gross tissue slice confirming T4 invasion.

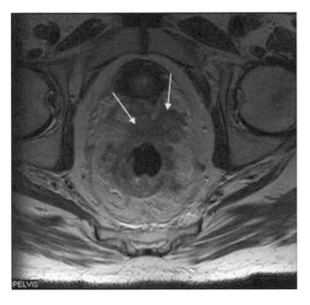

Figure 10.4   Axial T2-weighted image through a mid-rectal tumor. The tumor extends with a nodular infiltrative margin through and beyond Denonvilliers' fascia into the seminal vesicles indicating T4 disease (arrows).

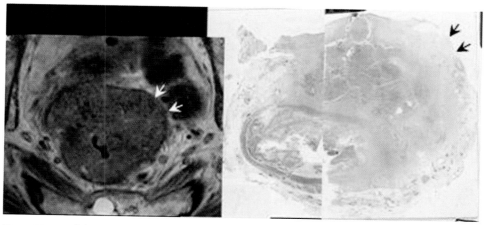

Figure 10.5   Axial T2-weighted image through a mid-rectal tumor, which is annular and extends through and beyond the muscle coat with a "pushing margin" and extends to the mesorectal margin (arrowheads). The corresponding histopathology section confirms margin involvement.

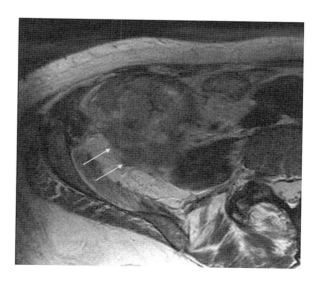

Figure 10.6   Axial T2-weighted image through an annular cecal tumor. There is evidence of tumor infiltration through and beyond the wall of the cecum posteriorly extending to the posterior parietal fascia and representing a potentially involved retroperitoneal surgical resection margin (arrows).

- Tumor is clear of the mesorectal fascia or the retroperitoneal surgical resection margins (Figure 10.5, Figure 10.6). In cases where tumor extends to or beyond the mesorectal or retroperitoneal fascia, conventional surgical approaches will result in cutting through tumor. In such cases, a more radical surgical approach is used and consideration is given to preoperative therapy aimed at downstaging the tumor.

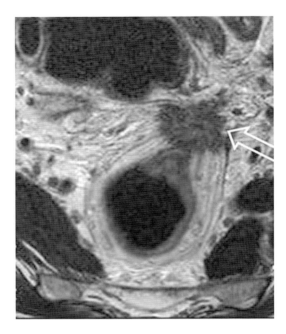

Figure 10.7   Axial T2-weighted image showing a peritoneal deposit (open arrow) in a patient with primary sigmoid adenocarcinoma.

- All sites of disease can be identified within the abdominal cavity and pelvis. Tumor deposits, e.g. peritoneal deposits or nodal disease in the pelvic sidewall or retroperitoneal should be identified preoperatively (Figure 10.7).

If any of the above features is present, then primary surgery will not be curative and more radical alternatives should be considered.

Anatomical considerations

The important anatomical structures are
1. the peritoneal reflection in relation to colon and rectum
2. the urogenital septum in the pelvis
3. the nerve plexuses within the pelvis
4. the mesocolon, mesorectum, mesorectal fascia, and retroperitoneal fascia.
5. the normal bowel wall.

Preoperative knowledge of the precise extent of spread in relation to these important anatomical structures is of potential importance in planning surgery as the surgical approach may be altered and this information may potentially influence the use of preoperative therapy.

(A)

(B)

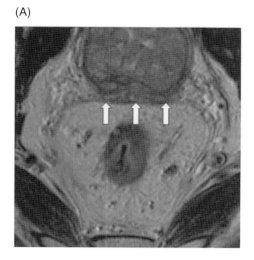
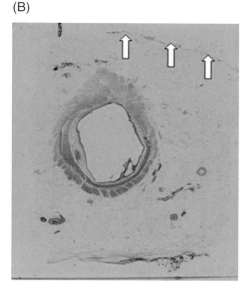

Figure 10.8   Axial T2-weighted image and corresponding histopathology section demonstrating Denonvilliers' fascia as a horizontal band of low signal intensity forming the anterior border of the mesorectal dissection (arrow).

The urogenital septum

Denonvilliers' fascia or the urogenital septum is an avascular sheath that originates from the embryonic pelvic floor. The structure serves to divide the posterior hindgut (rectum and perirectal structures) from the urogenital organs. Recent detailed embryological and anatomical studies have shown this to be present in both men and women [2]. It comprises collagenous and elastic fibers and smooth muscle cells mixed with nerve fibers that have their origins in the autonomic inferior hypogastric plexus. In the embryonic period, the septum is formed by a local condensation of mesenchymal connective tissue. In the male, this well-developed fascia produces a distinctive shiny anterior surface of the rectum (Denonvilliers fascia). In the female, it is termed as the "rectovaginal septum." In both sexes, it is visible on MRI as a low signal layer that can be traced up to the peritoneum superiorly (Figure 10.8) [3,4].

The pelvic nerve plexuses

The autonomic nerve supply to the pelvic viscera comes from two main sources. The sympathetic supply descends around the aorta and mingles at the origin of the

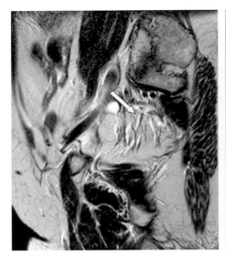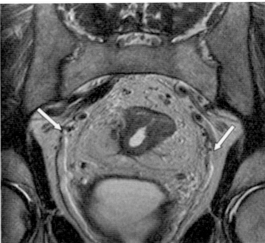

Figure 10.9 Sagittal MRI demonstrating the inferior hypogastric plexus (arrows). The plexus is also demonstrated on coronal imaging as beaded tubular structures of high signal intensity that lie in the para-sagittal plane.

inferior mesenteric artery, forming a superior hypogastric plexus just below the aortic bifurcation. The superior hypogastric plexus forms a wishbone and divides into two plexiform hypogastric nerves which descend 1–2 cm below each ureter to join the inferior hypogastric plexus. The hypogastric nerves are directly related to the retrorectal space, lying on the presacral fascia and often adherent to the visceral fascia when the rectum is pulled anteriorly. Care is required during pelvic dissection to preserve these nerves. The parasympathetic supply arises as the *nervi erigentes* from S_2, S_3, and S_4. They run laterally for 3 cm behind the parietal fascia before crossing it to join the inferior hypogastric plexus. The inferior hypogastric plexus lies sagittally. In the male, its mid-point is marked by the tip of the seminal vesicle, and in the female its anterior half lies against the upper third of the vagina. It lies in a plane medial to the vessels on the pelvic side wall. The plexus forms a lattice like meshwork up to 4 cm long in the sagittal plane and is readily visualized on MRI on parasagittal or paracoronal views (Figure 10.9).

The colonic mesentery and peritoneal coverings

Cecum and ascending colon

The cecum's and ascending colon's anterior, medial, lateral, and inferior walls are covered by serosa which is continuous with the parietal peritoneum. During

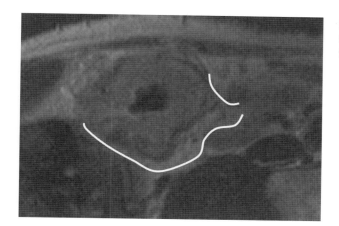

Figure 10.10 Axial MRI through the mid-abdomen demonstrating the transverse colon mesentery.

embryological development, the mesentery containing the ileocolic and right colic vessels becomes adherent to the posterior abdominal wall. The posterior area is devoid of serosa and is fused to the deep fascia of the posterior abdominal wall.

Transverse colon

The transverse colon is completely covered by serosa which continues as visceral peritoneum on either side of the transverse mesocolon. The transverse colon hangs freely on its mesentery which runs from the inferior pole of the right kidney across the second part of the duodenum and pancreas to the inferior pole of the left kidney (Figure 10.10).

Descending colon

Peritoneum covers the medial wall of the descending colon in continuity with the infracolic compartment and covers the anterior and lateral walls to reach the left paracolic gutter. As in the ascending colon, the rudimentary mesentery is fused to the posterior abdominal fascia (Figure 10.11).

Sigmoid colon

The sigmoid colon shares similarities to the transverse colon in that it is completely covered in peritoneum and hangs on a mesentery. Part of the posterior leaf of the sigmoid mesocolon is fused with the parietal peritoneum of the posterior abdominal wall (Figure 10.12).

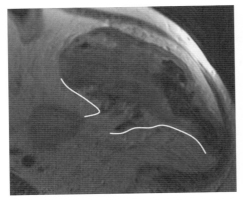

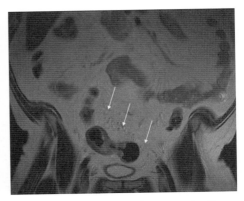

Figure 10.11 MRI and corresponding histopathology gross section demonstrating the rudimentary mesentery of the descending colon.

Figure 10.12 Sagittal MRI demonstrating the appearances of the sigmoid mesentery and lymphovascular drainage (arrows).

The mesorectum and peritoneal covering and mesorectal fascia

From the superior surface of the bladder, the peritoneum extends posteriorly to the sidewall of the pelvis. The peritoneum attaches as a V-shaped structure to the anterior 2/3 of the rectum.

The peritoneum-lined recess between the rectum and the posterior aspect of the bladder (or uterus) is the rectovesical or rectouterine pouch. On sagittal MR sections, the peritoneal reflection is demonstrated as a linear structure of low signal intensity that extends over the surface of the bladder and can be traced posteriorly to its point of attachment on the anterior aspect of the rectum (Figure 10.13).

The mesorectum is a distinct compartment that derives from the embryological hindgut and comprises a fatty layer of connective tissue and vessels and draining lymphatics that surrounds the rectum. It is covered by a distinct fascial covering derived from the visceral peritoneum – the mesorectal fascia. The mesorectal fascia is the glistening fascial layer enclosing the mesorectum, and thus anterior to the retrorectal space, variously named the visceral fascia of the mesorectum, fascia propria of the rectum, or presacral wing of the hypogastric sheath. The mesorectal fascia is demonstrated on axial sections as a low signal layer surrounding the mesorectum. This linear structure is demonstrated on cadaver axial MR images and correlated with the corresponding wholemount section as a distinct condensation of fascia encompassing the mesorectum and surrounded by loose areolar tissue. The mesorectal fascia is appreciated best on axial section and is seen as a low signal linear structure surrounding the mesorectum. It is consistently depicted on thin slice MR imaging (Figure 10.14).

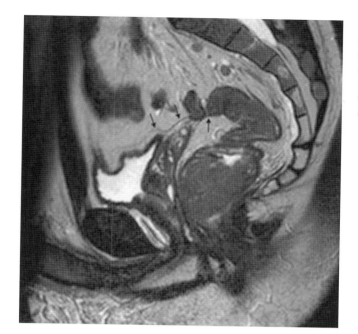

Figure 10.13   Sagittal MRI scan in a male patient, peritoneal reflection can be demonstrated as a low signal intensity line extending from the surface of the bladder to the anterior aspect of the rectum (arrows).

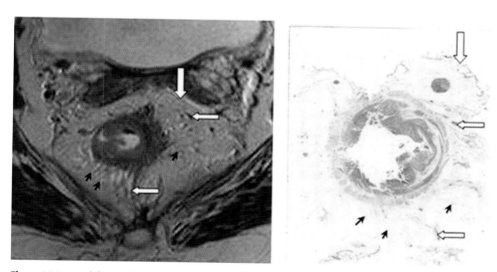

Figure 10.14   Axial T2-weighted image demonstrating the mesorectum and mesorectal fascia. The mesorectum is shown as a high signal intensity envelope (large arrow) surrounding the rectum. The mesorectum contains numerous vessels, lymphatics and lymph nodes (arrows), as well as small nerves giving it a rather complex structure. The interlacing connective tissue within the mesorectum is also demonstrated as low signal intensity strands (arrowheads).

(A)

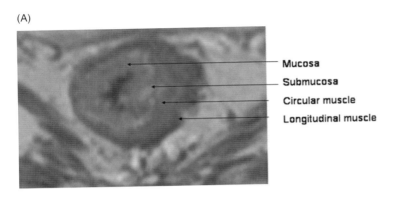

- Mucosa
- Submucosa
- Circular muscle
- Longitudinal muscle

(B)

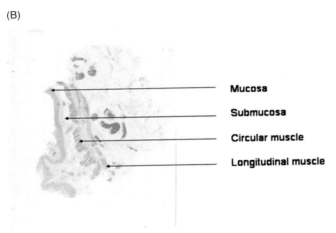

- Mucosa
- Submucosa
- Circular muscle
- Longitudinal muscle

Figure 10.15   Axial T2-weighted image demonstrating the bowel wall layers. The mucosa is demonstrated as low signal intensity and is only 1 mm or so thick and may not be seen on routine MRI images. The submucosa is routinely demonstrated and is seen as high signal intensity and the muscularis propria formed by the circular and longitudinal muscle coats are demonstrated (arrows).

The mesorectum is demonstrated as a high signal intensity (fat signal) envelope surrounding the rectum containing vessels which are depicted as low signal (owing to signal void produced by blood flow), and lymph nodes are shown as high signal (owing to high fluid content) ovoid structures. Small nerves within the mesorectum are not visualized but interlacing connective tissue within the mesorectum is shown as low signal intensity strands.

The normal bowel wall

In cross section, the rectal wall comprises the mucosal layer, the muscularis mucosae, submucosa, and the muscularis propria which in turn comprises the circular and outer longitudinal layers. The two layers are separated by a thin layer of connective tissue containing the neuromyenteric plexus.

The MRI appearances of the bowel wall show the mucosal layer as a fine low signal intensity line with the thicker higher signal submucosal layer lying beneath this. The muscularis propria can sometimes be depicted as two distinct layers: the inner circular layer and the outer longitudinal layer. The outer muscle layer has an irregular corrugated appearance and there are frequently interruptions within this layer owing to vessels entering the rectal wall. The perirectal fat appears as high signal surrounding the low signal of the muscularis propria (Figure 10.15).

Tumor morphology and T staging

The spectrum of morphologic subtypes demonstrated on MR imaging and histology sections reflect the stages of development of invasive carcinoma, and an understanding of the tumor morphology greatly assists in the interpretation of in vivo imaging and T staging. Tumors of the colon and rectum generally develop as a consequence of malignant change within a polyp or sessile plaque and then may enlarge and ulcerate centrally.

The vast majority of colorectal cancers are moderately differentiated adenocarcinomas – 20% are well-differentiated and approximately 20% are poorly differentiated [5]. Most tumors are believed to arise from pre-existing mucosal adenomas and exhibit varying degrees of dysplasia from mild to severe. Adenomas may be polypoid or flat and have either a tubular or a villous configuration. The development of carcinoma in such lesions is characterized by the ability to invade the submucosa. As tumors become more aggressive, they invade the deeper layers of the bowel wall and beyond, and develop the capacity for lymphatic and vascular invasion.

Annular and semiannular tumors

The most common macroscopic appearance is that of an ulcerating tumor with a central depression and raised rolled edges. This feature can be readily recognized on high resolution imaging using MRI. In less advanced cases, an elevated plaque

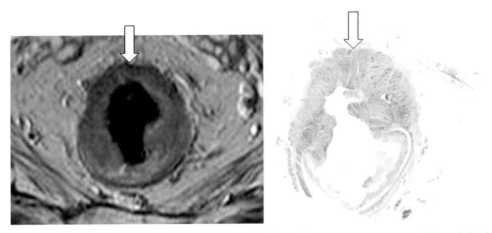

Figure 10.16   Typical appearance of adenocarcinoma of the colon or rectum. Here, an axial T2-weighted image demonstrating an annular tumor with a central depression representing central ulceration and corresponding to the most invasive portion of the tumor (arrow).

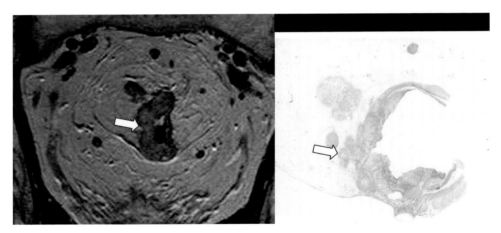

Figure 10.17   Adenocarcinoma with deep central ulceration. Here, a more infiltrating tumor is demonstrated with erosion at the base of the tumor representing the central ulcer which forms the infiltrating margin of the tumor (arrow).

of intermediate signal intensity projects into the lumen forming a U-shaped thickened disc that corresponds to a semiannular plaque of tumor on histology sections (Figure 10.16).

As tumors advance, this plaque shows a central depression forming a mass with a central ulcerating section that corresponds to the most invasive portion of the tumor (Figure 10.17).

(A)

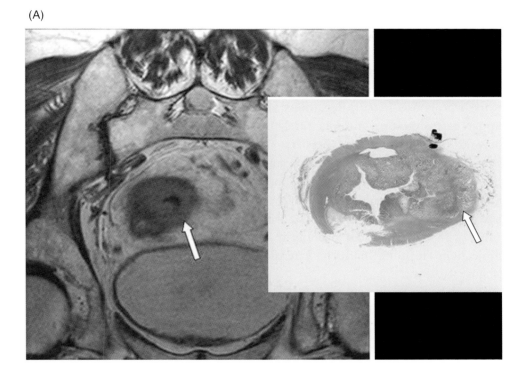

(B)

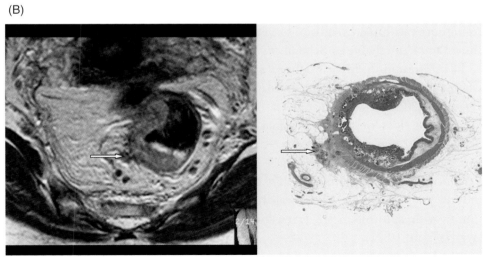

Figure 10.18   (A) Semi-annular tumor with a well-circumscribed "pushing" advancing margin top
(arrow) (B) bottom, a tumor with nodular infiltrating margins (arrow).

When rectal tumors invade through the bowel wall into perirectal fat, they commonly do so with a well-circumscribed margin. In some cases however, the pattern of spread is widely infiltrative with ill-defined borders. Malignant epithelium dissects between normal structures so that no distinct border to the tumor can be identified, and this pattern of spread has long been known to worsen prognosis [5,6,7]. Regardless of differentiation, colorectal tumors unlike upper gastrointestinal tumors rarely show submucosal or intramural spread beyond their macroscopic borders. This characteristic is important in the surgical planning of distal resection margins [8,9,10]. These two histopathology patterns are demonstrable on MR images and can thus be used as criteria for identifying T3 spread into perirectal or pericolonic fat. Tumor extension beyond the bowel wall is manifested as intermediate signal intensity spreading either with a broad-based pushing margin (Figure 10.18A) or with finger-like projections forming nodular extensions into perirectal or pericolonic fat (Figure 10.18B).

Spiculation, on the other hand, has been described as a manifestation of tumor spread into fat but when this appearance on MR images is compared with corresponding histology sections, this represents perivascular cuffing and peritumoral spicules of connective tissue that do not contain tumor (Figure 10.19). Similarly, the usefulness of irregularity of the bowel wall is also limited as this frequently correlates with normal bowel contour made irregular by corrugated and sometimes incomplete bands of longitudinal muscle. This criterion has also been shown to be unreliable by Schnall et al. [11].

T1 infiltration on MRI is defined as preservation of the submucosal layer and when this is present, it is a helpful feature with high positive predictive value (Figure 10.20).

However, loss of the high signal mucosal layer will not allow distinction between a T1 and a T2 lesion since microscopic infiltration into circular muscle (pT2) has an identical appearance on MRI as complete replacement of the submucosal layer by tumor (pT1). By the same analogy, a tumor occupying the full thickness of the bowel wall (pT2) can be difficult to distinguish from a tumor with sub-millimetre extension through the outer longitudinal muscle layer (Figure 10.21).

When colorectal adenocarcinomas encompass the full circumference of the bowel wall forming an annular growth, they produce marked narrowing of the bowel lumen increasing the risk of bowel obstruction or perforation. Tumors may also ulcerate despite their relatively small size: the ulcerating stricture may also

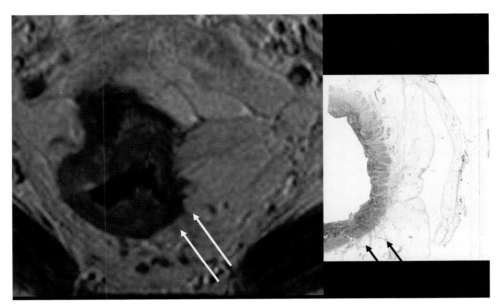

Figure 10.19   Axial imaging demonstrating speculation. The fine low signal intensity strands demonstrated in the perirectal tissues are a feature of desmoplasia rather than tumor infiltration (arrows).

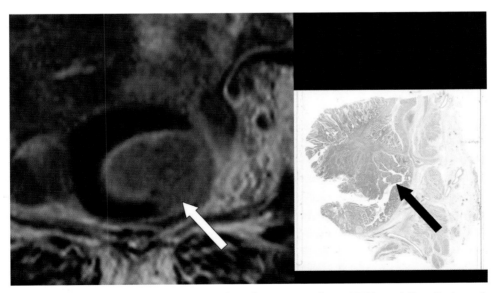

Figure 10.20   This is an axial T2-weight image through a stage T1 polyp on MRI (arrow). Here, the tumor is confined to the superficial layers and no deep infiltration is demonstrated. The submucosal layer can be demonstrated as a separate layer deep to the intermediate signal intensity of the superficial tumor.

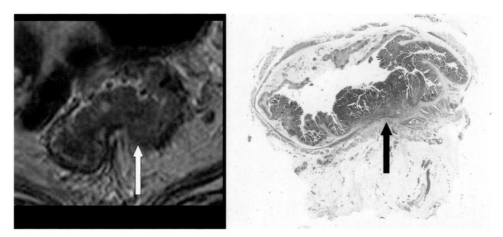

Figure 10.21   Typical appearance of a T2 tumor. Here, tumor extends to involve the full thickness of the submucosa, and there is effacement of the muscularis propria layer indicating likely T2 infiltration.

produce stenosis. Central ulceration of tumor causes focal thinning and stricturing of the bowel wall. On occasion, severe ulceration by the tumor will cause more diffuse thinning of the bowel so that the bowel layers are no longer discernible. Ulcerating tumors are the most difficult to delineate on MR images, showing little or no tumor bulk but conversely demonstrate thinning of the bowel wall layers making individual layers difficult to differentiate, and thus the degree of extra-mural spread is poorly depicted (Figure 10.22).

Polypoidal tumors

Exophytic or polypoidal tumors have a pronounced protuberant appearance with the tumor mass projecting into the lumen. A number of studies have observed that such polypoidal lesions are often of a relatively low grade of malignancy despite forming large protuberant and even obstructing intraluminal mass lesions [12,13,14]. Early tumors developing within benign polypoidal adenomas usually become pedunculated, and are broken into lobules with intercommunicating clefts resulting in a characteristic papillary surface. One such form is the villous adeno-carcinoma, which presents typically as a protuberant soft and often friable sessile mass with a shaggy or velvety surface. Such tumors can attain a large size with only minimal infiltration of the bowel wall.

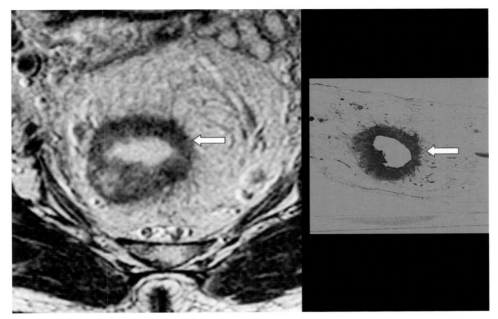

Figure 10.22   Ulcerating tumor. Here, there has been a total destruction of the bowel wall layers with erosion and thinning of the muscularis propria caused by an ulcerating tumor (arrow).

On MRI, these tumors project into the lumen as a rounded protuberant mass.

Since many of these polyps are at an early stage, a preserved high signal intensity corresponding to a partially preserved submucosal layer is often shown deep to the polyp. The surface of these polypoidal tumor mass lesions frequently shows clefts containing high signal corresponding to mucous fluid on the papillary or frond-like tumor surface (Figure 10.23).

Mucinous tumors

Mucinous tumors form a distinct morphological subgroup characterized by their gelatinous appearance caused by secretion of mucus by the tumor cells. These account for 10% of carcinomas of the large intestine and appear to represent a poor prognostic subgroup. The term "mucinous" is strictly defined as tumor containing > 75% mucin [15]. A number of authors have observed the association between mucinous carcinoma and poor prognosis [15,16] which is thought to relate to the fact that these tumors have a poorly defined advancing margin and are often very advanced at presentation [17]. They are also thought to infiltrate diffusely and unlike non-

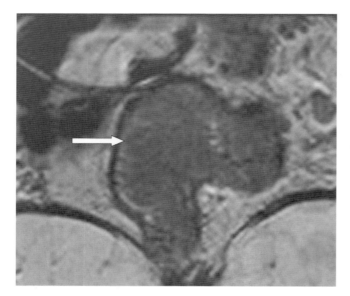

Figure 10.23 Polypoidal tumor. Axial T2-weighted image showing a typical appearance of a polypoidal tumor. Here, a protuberant mass is demonstrated, often with surface clefts indicating a papillary surface in keeping with a polypoidal mass.

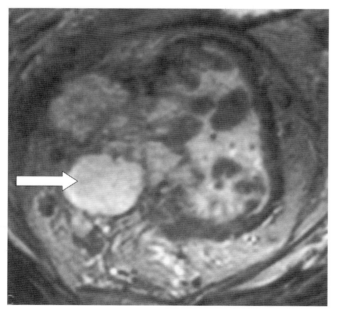

Figure 10.24 A typical appearance of mucinous tumor (arrow). Focal high signal intensity is demonstrated within the tumor although some intermediate signal intensity is shown indicating that this contains mucin. This appearance can be confused with perforation, but the presence of intermediate signal intensity within these high signal intensity pools is more in keeping with mucinous tumor.

mucinous tumors, they can spread intramurally. On MRI, this form of tumor is of very high signal intensity (same signal as water). Their diffusely infiltrating nature often results in preservation of anatomical layers so that the bowel wall layers sometimes show expansion by high signal intensity (Figure 10.24).

Staging colonic and rectal tumors

The extent of local spread

Dukes' [18] paper highlighted the importance of extent of extramural spread in the prediction of local recurrence as well as survival. Survival figures for tumors extending beyond the bowel wall were 89.7% for slight spread, 80% for moderate spread, and 57% for extensive spread. The measurement is taken from the outer edge of the longitudinal muscle layer. Importantly, Dukes also observed that once spread beyond the bowel wall occurs, the incidence of lymph node invasion increases rising from 14.2% in tumors confined to the bowel wall to 43.2% in those tumors extending beyond the bowel wall. Pathologists have long recognized that with increasing depth of spread, there is an increasing incidence of nodal involvement and extramural venous invasion [5,19,20]. Thus, these tumors frequently represent the poorest end of the prognostic spectrum and are at very high risk of both local and distant failure.

The depth of tumor spread is measured from the outer muscle coat to the outermost edge of intermediate signal intensity tumor.

Image interpretation criteria for T staging

Criteria for identifying the layers of the bowel wall and T staging tumor were originally proposed from work using the endoluminal coil [21,22,23,24]. However, these studied small groups of patients, and both the image interpretation criteria and image acquisition parameters were not consistent. In particular, the observation by Schnall et al. [11] that "non-luminal irregularity" was an unreliable sign of T3 tumor contradicted observations made by Murano et al. [21], Joosten et al. [22], Pegios et al. [23], and Vogl et al. [24] that irregularity and spiculation of the outer margins of the muscularis propria indicated tumor infiltration into perirectal fat. In addition, Pegios et al. [23] and Vogl et al. [24] suggested that intravenous contrast enhancement was useful in identifying tumors with spread beyond the bowel wall. Conversely, Okizuka [25] showed that intravenous contrast enhancement resulted in overstaging owing to perirectal vessel enhancement. Despite these inconsistencies, most authors however agreed that compared with T1 weighted images, T2 weighted images permitted the best contrast between tumor and the bowel wall and accuracies of 80% or above were achieved using the endoluminal coil. Unfortunately, endoluminal techniques are not generally feasible as a staging

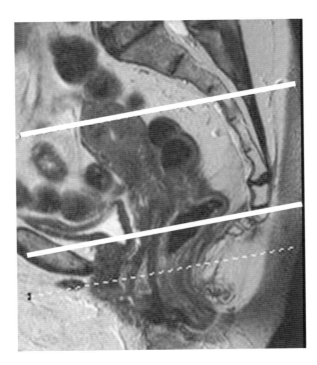

Figure 10.25 High-resolution image technique. Oblique axial images are obtained orthogonal to the rectal wall as shown in order to obtain a true axial image of the primary tumor.

method in colorectal cancer since stenosis, stricturing, pain and discomfort, bowel wall motion, inaccessibility of colonic and rectal lesions above the distal 10 cm of rectum, and coil migration all make consistent acquisition of good quality images very difficult.

The initial sequences performed are the localization images, in the coronal and sagittal planes, to image the tumor and plan the high-resolution images that are performed axial to the rectum.

• The first series is the sagittal T2W-FSE, which enables identification of the primary tumor.
• The second series – large field of view axial sections of the whole pelvis from the iliac crest to the symphysis pubis.
• While the second series is being acquired, the high-resolution images can be planned (Figure 10.25).
• The sagittal T2-weighted images obtained are used to plan T2-weighted thin-section axial images through the rectal cancer and adjacent perirectal tissues. It is critical that these images are performed perpendicular to the long-axis of the rectum. The images are obtained by using a 16-cm field of view and 3-mm section thickness.

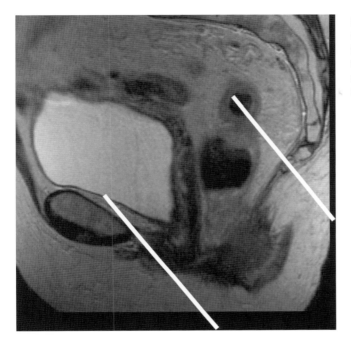

Figure 10.26 Sagittal scan showing the planning planes for coronal imaging of low tumors in order to demonstrate the anal canal most optimally.

- The rapid change in caliber of the rectal lumen at the level of the anorectal junction limits the usefulness of oblique axial imaging alone. At this level, axial images may not show the rectal wall in its entirety, and clear delineation between the outer edge of the rectal wall and the levator muscle may not be possible. This can potentially lead to overstaging. It is therefore useful to utilize a high spatial resolution coronal imaging sequence which will show the levator, the sphincter complex, the intersphincteric plane, and the relationship to the rectal wall most optimally (Figure 10.26).

From observation of features described above and from published image interpretation criteria, the T stage can be predicted.

The demonstration of intermediate signal intensity within the mucosa and submucosa with preservation of a thin layer of submucosa deep to "tumor" signal corresponds to tumor confined to the submucosa (pT1) tumor. When tumor signal extends into the circular muscle coat but does not extend through the full thickness of muscle, this corresponds to histological pT2. However, when the full thickness of muscle coat appears to be replaced by intermediate signal intensity, this corresponds to pT2 or pT3 tumor and it is often not possible to distinguish between the two (Figure 10.27).

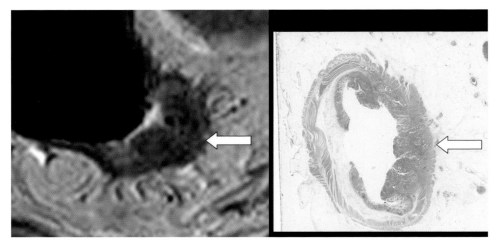

Figure 10.27   Borderline T2/T3 tumor. Axial scans showing semiannular tumor infiltrating through the full thickness of the muscularis propria (arrow). It can be difficult to judge whether the muscularis propria is completely intact. Therefore, the distinction between T2 and T3 tumors, when there is less than 1 mm of spread beyond the muscularis propria, can be difficult.

A broad-based pushing margin of intermediate signal intensity extending into perirectal or pericolonic fat corresponds to pT3 tumor, and the more infiltrative form shows finger-like nodular extension of tumor into perirectal/pericolonic fat which is thought to have unfavorable prognosis.

The bowel contour will often show an irregular contour and when this is compared with the corresponding histology sections, it can be seen that this irregularity is because of the normal corrugated appearance of this muscle coat.

Fine spicules of low signal intensity are sometimes seen radiating from the bowel wall into adjacent fat. In some cases, this corresponds to florid perivascular cuffing of connective tissue; in other cases, this is because of peritumoral desmoplastic response. It is a very unreliable feature of T3 spread.

Within each T stage, there is heterogeneity of survival and there has been much interest in identifying poor prognostic groups within each stage. Both T1 and T2 tumors have a very high 5-year survival but the widest range in survival is demonstrated in patients with T3 tumors. For example, a T3 tumor with only 1–2 mm of extramural spread has an identical prognosis to T2 tumors [26]. A number of authors have shown a relationship between poor survival and increasing depth of extramural spread that is independent of other prognostic factors including the circumferential margin status [27,28]. It is therefore worth noting that although the accuracy of preoperative staging techniques is limited by overstaging or understaging of borderline T3/T2 tumors, there is rather limited importance in differentiating between minimal T3 infiltration and T2 lesions since both have favorable survival and are thus unlikely to obtain benefit from adjuvant therapy unless the potential circumferential margin is threatened. Conversely, the successful identification of tumors with increasing extramural spread is of great importance as histopathology studies have shown poor survival in this group of patients. In our experience, the majority of patients with tumor infiltrating 5 mm or more beyond the muscularis propria are correctly identified, and extramural depth, as measured using MRI, shows direct agreement with corresponding histopathological measurements [29,30].

Spread beyond the peritoneal membrane

This is defined as perforation of the peritoneal membrane by tumor and the consequent spillage of tumor cells is presumed to result in both local recurrence and transcoelomic dissemination. Local peritoneal involvement was detected in 25.8% (54/209) of cases. This is an independent prognostic factor and predicts for local recurrence after surgery for colorectal cancers [31,32].

Colonic T4 disease is classified histologically as tumor involving the free peritoneal cavity or invading other organs. On MRI definition, this can be defined as perforation of tumor signal through the peritoneal covering of the bowel wall or penetration of adjacent structures. As a consequence, images should be interpreted with knowledge of peritoneal anatomy and an understanding of the peritonealized vs. non-peritonealized surfaces of the colon and rectum (Figure 10.28).

The transverse and sigmoid colon are almost completely invested in peritoneum, so any tumor breach that extends through the bowel wall away from the sigmoid mesocolon will be defined as T4 disease (Figure 10.29).

Whilst tumors of the cecum, ascending, and descending colon will perforate through a peritonealized surface anteriorly, posteriorly the colon is non-peritonealized and therefore cannot be T4 disease unless the tumor has penetrated adjacent organs such as the kidneys or duodenum (Figure 10.30).

The anterior wall of the upper rectum is covered by the peritoneal reflection, and transcoelomic spread with disseminated intra-abdominal disease will occur if there is ulceration through the peritoneum [32]. Obvious tumor spread through and beyond the peritoneal reflection can be readily identified (Figure 10.31).

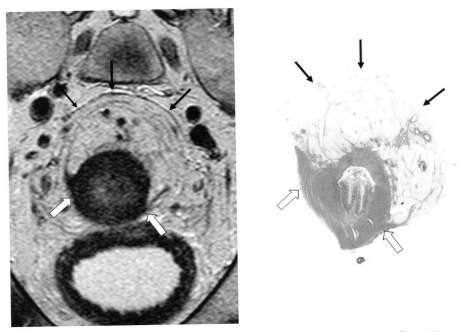

Figure 10.28   Axial MR image through the upper third of the rectum and corresponding TME specimen illustrating the peritonealized (open arrow) vs. non-peritonealized (black arrows) surfaces of the rectum.

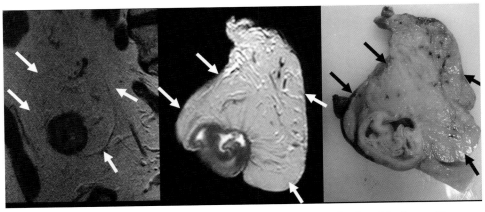

Figure 10.29   MR image and histopathology specimen image showing the sigmoid colon and its peritoneal covering (arrow).

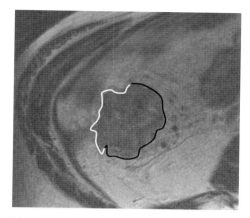

Figure 10.30   MR axial image showing a cecal tumor and the peritonealized surface (outlined white) and non-peritonealized (outlined black) surface.

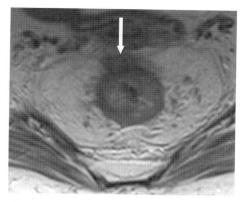

Figure 10.31   Oblique axial image through an upper third rectal tumor. There is tumor extension through and beyond the peritonealized surface indicating T4 infiltration (arrow).

However, cases will be missed by MRI owing to failure to resolve microscopic infiltration of peritoneal-lined clefts. Radiologists should be prompted to search for subtle features of peritoneal perforation where tumors appear to lie in contact with a peritonealized surface. Characteristically, this manifests as nodular extension of tumor through the peritoneal reflection and is best demonstrated on axial high-resolution images performed perpendicular to the peritoneal attachment.

Lymph node spread

Dukes and Bussey [33] first noted the relationship between the number of involved nodes and 5-year survival, showing that for 1, 2–5, 6–10, and more than 10 affected nodes, the 5-year survival rates were 63.6%, 36.1%, 21.9%, and 2.1%, respectively [33]. This observation was reaffirmed [5,34,35]. These authors have shown that if four or more nodes are involved by tumor, survival is significantly worsened, illustrating the importance of ensuring adequate node sampling through meticulous lymph node dissection [36].

In preoperative assessment of lymph node status, the following features need to be taken into account:

The total number of nodes involved worsens prognosis particularly when four or more nodes are involved; therefore, the preoperative identification of such patients can be an indication for preoperative therapy [37,38].

The presence of tumor containing lymph nodes close to the surgical resection margin increases the risk of recurrence [39]. This certainly applies to nodes that appear obviously replaced by tumor and with extracapsular extension. In these cases, tumor will be present on the circumferential surface of the excised specimen and preoperative therapy is required. There is no data to show that there is a risk of local recurrence in patients with nodes that are fully encapsulated (morphologically normal on MRI), so the role of preoperative therapy in such cases is less well established.

In Japan, patients with nodes lying outside the mesorectal fascia in rectal cancers may be treated by extended lymphadenectomy in order to achieve clearance of tumor [40,41,42]; those that remain unresected may be responsible for local recurrence despite apparently clear surgical resection margins [43]. In Europe, patients with nodal disease in this compartment do not routinely undergo pelvic sidewall dissection and preoperative therapy is usually given instead [44].

The ability to determine reliably node-negative status preoperatively could result in less aggressive surgery and preoperative therapy in some patients. At present, preoperative imaging cannot reliably exclude microscopic nodal involvement, and the decision to treat using local excision should be based on histological assessment of the depth of tumor invasion [45,46].

It is widely accepted that using size criteria alone will result in false-positive diagnosis and this is supported by histological studies. For example, in a survey of over 12 000 lymph nodes in rectal cancer, Dworak showed considerable size overlap between normal or reactive nodes and those containing metastases [47]. He found that the only positive lymph nodes in 31 out of 98 rectal cancer patients measured < 5 mm. Schnall et al., [11] using endorectal MR, noted that positive lymph nodes varied substantially in size, with 5 out of 12 nodes measuring 5 mm or less containing tumor [11].

The internal architecture of nodes has been studied using endoluminal ultrasound [48,49]. These studies showed that the internal texture of an imaged node may correlate better with the presence of metastasis than nodal size, and that inhomogeneity and hilar reflectivity are important discriminators of nodal status [50]. It has been noted that the specificity of endoluminal ultrasound (EUS) could be improved if the echogenicity of a node was considered in addition to its size; metastases were commoner in nodes of mixed intranodal echogenicity than in those of uniform hyperechogenicity. The signal intensity and border characteristics of lymph nodes have been compared with nodal size as predictors of final nodal stage. In a study in rectal cancer on MRI have also been evaluated. In study correlating lymph nodes on MRI with pathology from 42 consecutive patients undergoing TME surgery, 437 lymph nodes were harvested [51]. Of these, 102, all < 3 mm in diameter, were not identified on MR images (two contained metastases) and a further 51 were outside the field of view imaged at high resolution. Two hundred and eighty-four lymph nodes were then compared with histopathology. The size of lymph nodes containing metastases in MR images varied greatly and 58% of positive nodes were less than 5 mm in diameter. MR measurement of nodal diameters ranged from 2 mm to 10 mm in 119 benign nodes from 20 node-negative patients and from 3 mm to 15 mm in 60 positive nodes from 22 node-positive patients. Furthermore, in 71% patients with lymph node metastases the size of normal or reactive nodes was similar to or greater than the smallest positive node in the same specimen. Whatever size cut-off used, the overall predictive value of MR size was poor because of substantial overlap in size between nodes that are benign and malignant.

When signal intensity of nodes were evaluated in this study, only 4% of high signal intensity nodes were malignant on MRI, 19% of nodes that appeared to be of the same signal intensity as the primary tumor were malignant and only 13% of low signal intensity were malignant. On the other hand, 91% of nodes containing foci of different signal intensities present within the node were malignant. Therefore, using mixed signal intensity as a marker for nodal involvement gave a sensitivity of only 48% but a high specificity, 98.6%. We observed that mixed MR signal intensity usually corresponded to tumor deposits with areas of necrosis or extra-cellular mucin pools (Figure 10.32) histologically.

Evaluation of the border contour of lymph nodes was also a good predictor of nodal status; only 6% of nodes with smooth borders contained metastases compared with 92% with irregular borders (example shown in Figure 10.33), giving a sensitivity of 75% and a specificity of 98%.

Thus, virtually all normal or reactive lymph nodes were characterized by uniform signal intensity and smooth, sharply demarcated borders. In many nodes, it was possible to demonstrate a low signal rim surrounding the node which represented the lymph node capsule; in addition the afferent and efferent lymphatic channels could sometimes be seen (Figure 10.34).

Fifty-seven percent of nodes with an irregular border were completely replaced by tumor with no visible lymphoid tissue present (all > 3 mm in diameter). When lymph node border and intensity were combined, the sensitivity and specificity were optimized. Metastases were demonstrated in nearly all lymph nodes with either an irregular border or a mixed intensity signal, and only a small percentage of nodes with smooth borders and a uniform signal contained metastases.

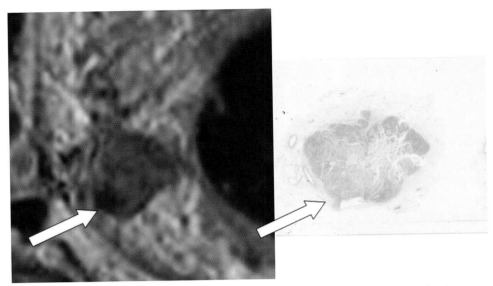

Figure 10.32 MR and corresponding histopathology H + E stained section of a lymph node. The MR shows a lymph node containing mixed foci of signal intensity. The corresponding histopathology section shows this mixed signal intensity correspond to tumor and foci of tumor necrosis (arrow).

Micrometastatic disease defined as tumor foci < 2 mm within lymph nodes could not be identified.

The inability to identify nodes < 5 mm in diameter is recognized as a significant limitation of staging by EUS [52], with only 13% of positive lymph nodes measuring < 5 mm in diameter being detected in one series [53]. Using high-resolution techniques many nodes measuring 2–5 mm are identified. Whilst the ability of MRI to resolve nodes < 3 mm in diameter is suboptimal, it would seem that MR evaluation of nodes using these morphological criteria will result in understaging of very few patients. The quality of high-resolution imaging is critical in being able to resolve and characterize these nodes, and viewing the zoomed images on a workstation is recommended. In cases where image degradation has occurred owing to patient movement or if there is a poor signal to noise ratio, confident assessment of nodal status will be limited.

Venous spread

Talbot and Ritchie (1980) [54] published a histological analysis of 703 rectal cancer surgical specimens. They observed that the presence of invasion of extramural

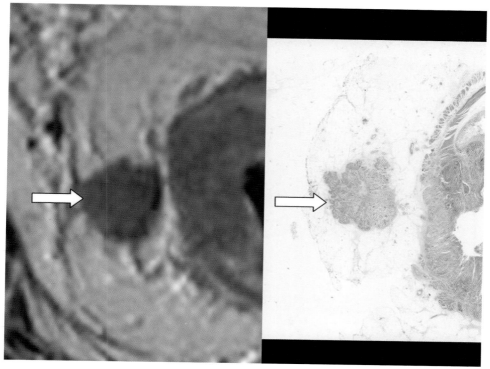

Figure 10.33   MR and corresponding histopathology H + E stained section of a lymph node. The MR shows a lymph node with an irregular border (arrow). The corresponding histopathology section shows this irregular border corresponds to tumor breach of the lymph node capsule.

veins by tumor was associated with a low 5-year survival rate (33%), and was an important prognostic factor associated with a much lower survival regardless of Dukes stage. In subsequent studies, the presence of venous invasion was correlated with survival and the pattern of treatment failure [55,56]. Venous invasion predicted significantly reduced actuarial survival rates in patients with node-negative tumors. Furthermore, when extramural venous invasion was demonstrated (present in 22% of specimens), there was a significant decrease in distant recurrence-free 5-year survival. Venous invasion was thus shown as not only a poor predictor of survival but also the third strongest independent predictor of metastasis, after lymph node status and extent of local tumor infiltration. Harrison *et al.* [19] reaffirmed this observation showing an improved 5-year survival rate associated with absence of extramural vein invasion by tumor, which retained independent prognostic significance after multivariate analysis of 12 pathological variables. Even in patients

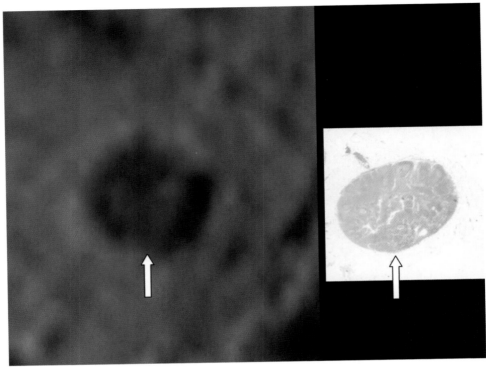

Figure 10.34   MR and corresponding histopathology H + E stained section of a normal lymph node. Note that the lymph node capsule, efferent and afferent lymphatic channels can be visualized (arrow).

undergoing careful radical excision of the rectum and mesorectum, venous invasion remains an important independent prognostic factor [57,58]. By careful correlation with histopathology specimens we have shown that high-resolution MRI can identify extramural vascular invasion (EMVI) preoperatively [29] and we have also demonstrated that preoperative MRI predicts postoperative histological EMVI with 80% accuracy, and that the presence or absence of this particular feature can be used to stratify patients into clearly separate prognostic groups. Patients diagnosed with MRI-EMVI positive tumors have a significantly worse outcome with an overall risk of developing distant metastases (either synchronous or delayed) greater than 50%, compared with only 12% for patients who are MRI-EMVI negative. Extramural venous invasion is recognized on MRI by characteristic serpiginous extension of tumor signal into perirectal or pericolonic fat (Figure 10.35) [29].

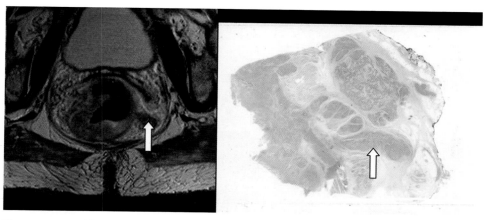

Figure 10.35   Axial MR of colonic tumor and rectal tumor showing extramural venous invasion with histopathological correlation (arrow).

The circumferential resection margin in colon and rectal cancer

Rectal cancer

The mesorectal fascia represents the potential CRM in patients undergoing TME surgery and its clear demonstration on MRI enables prediction of final CRM status in patients undergoing TME surgery. We define potential CRM involvement if tumor extends to within 1 mm of the mesorectal fascia on MR images. Hall *et al.* [59] prospectively studied outcome in patients with positive circumferential margins. In contrast to the group's earlier studies carried out in non-TME specimens [60,61], positive CRM did not predict local recurrence but did influence overall disease-free interval and survival rates. It was postulated therefore that CRM positive status following TME surgery might either reflect poor surgical clearance or advanced disease that cannot be influenced by meticulous surgery. Our observation that tumors with positive CRM status had more extensive local spread than tumors with negative CRM status suggests that the latter is an important contributing factor to positive CRM status. It also suggests that this group of patients could potentially benefit from therapy that causes tumor regression away from the potential CRM. Since the mandatory discussion of staging investigations including high-resolution MR staging of rectal tumors has become our policy, we have observed a substantial fall in CRM involvement. National guidelines indicate a rate of 20% or less as acceptable, but with the use of preoperative downstaging chemoradiotherapy, resection margin involvement rates of < 5% are achievable.

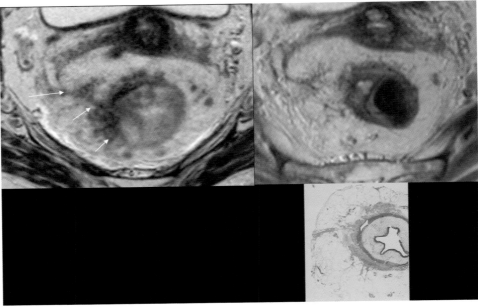

Figure 10.36   Axial MRI showing locally advanced rectal primary, nodular tumor extends to the potential surgical circumferential resection margin (arrow). This patient was given preoperative neoadjuvant chemotherapy followed by chemoradiotherapy. The posttreatment MRI shows tumor regression away from the surgical circumferential resection margin. The corresponding postsurgical TME specimen shows that there has been tumor regression and no tumor is present at the margins.

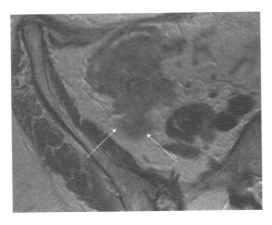

Figure 10.37   Axial MRI showing locally advanced colonic tumor. Infiltrating tumor extends posteriorly to the potential retroperitoneal surgical margin (arrows). Following surgery, the resected specimen shows extensive tumor posteriorly with involvement of the circumferential resection margin.

When a negative CRM is achieved, this reduces the risk of local recurrence and improves overall survival (Figure 10.36) [62]. It is hoped that in future, similarly aggressive but selective preoperative treatment strategies may be applied for colonic tumors [63].

Imaging of the colonic resection margin (RSM)

The retroperitoneal surgical resection margin is the "bare area" or non-peritonea-lized fascia which forms the plane of dissection for tumors of the cecum, ascending, and descending colon. Resection margin involvement has been shown to occur almost exclusively when the tumor is invading through the posterior wall of the distal cecum or the proximal ascending colon. The frequency of RSM involvement is thought to be approximately 7% which coincides with the 10% rate of local recurrence after right hemicolectomy [64]. Preoperative imaging should therefore identify those posterior cecal and ascending colon tumors that appear too close to the posterior fascia. Such tumors should be considered at risk of RSM involvement (Figure 10.37).

REFERENCES

1. Burton, S., Brown, G., Daniels, I. R., *et al*. MRI directed multidisciplinary team preoperative treatment strategy: the way to eliminate positive circumferential margins? *Br J Cancer*, **94**:3 (2006), 351–7.

2. Aigner, F., Zbar, A. P., Ludwikowski, B., *et al*. The rectogenital septum: morphology, function, and clinical relevance. *Dis Colon Rectum*, **47**:2 (2004), 131–40.

3. Heald, R. J., Moran, B. J., Brown, G., and Daniels, I. Optimal Total mesorectal excision for rectal cancer is in front of Denonvilliers Fascia. *Br J Surg*, **91**:1 (2004), 121–3.

4. Brown, G., Kirkham, A., Williams, G. T., *et al*. High-resolution MRI of the anatomy important in total mesorectal excision of the rectum. *AJR Am J Roentgenol*, **182**:2 (2004), 431–9.

5. Jass, J. R., Atkin, W. S., Cuzick, J., *et al*. The grading of rectal cancer: historical perspectives and a multivariate analysis of 447 cases. *Histopathology*, **10**:5 (1986), 437–59.

6. Grinnell, R. S. The grading and prognosis of carcinoma of the colon and rectum. *Ann Surg*, **109** (1939), 500–33.

7. Spratt, J. A. and Spjut, H. J. Prevalence and prognosis of carcinoma of the colon and rectum. *Cancer*, **20** (1967), 1976–85.

8. Andreola, S., Leo, E., Belli, F., Lavarino, C., Bufalino, R., Tomasic, G., Baldini, M. T., Valvo, F., Navarria, P., and Lombardi, F. Distal intramural spread in adenocarcinoma of the lower third of the rectum treated with total rectal resection and coloanal anastomosis. *Dis Colon Rectum*, **40**:1 (1997), 25–9.

9. Hughes, T. G., Jenevein, E. P., and Poulos, E. Intramural spread of colon carcinoma. A pathologic study. *Am J Surg*, **146**:6 (1983), 697–9.

10. Madsen, P. M. and Christiansen, J. Distal intramural spread of rectal carcinomas. *Dis Colon Rectum*, **29**:4 (1986), 279–82.

11. Schnall, M. D., Furth, E. E., Rosato, E. F., and Kressel, H. Y. Rectal tumor stage: correlation of endorectal MR imaging and pathologic findings. *Radiology*, **190**:3 (1994), 709–14.

12. Cohen, A. M., Wood, W. C., Gunderson, L. L., and Shinnar, M. Pathological studies in rectal cancer. *Cancer*, **45**:12 (1980), 2965–8.

13. Bjerkeset, T., Morild, I., Mork, S., and Soreide, O. Tumor characteristics in colorectal cancer and their relationship to treatment and prognosis. *Dis Colon Rectum*, **30**:12 (1987), 934–8.

14. Michelassi, F., Vannucci, L., Montag, A., *et al.* Importance of tumor morphology for the long term prognosis of rectal adenocarcinoma. *Am Surg*, **54**:6 (1988), 376–9.

15. Sasaki, O., Atkin, W. S., and Jass, J. R. Mucinous carcinoma of the rectum. *Histopathology*, **11**:3 (1987), 259–72.

16. Pihl, E., Nairn, R. C., Hughes, E. S., Cuthbertson, A. M., and Rollo A. J. Mucinous colorectal carcinoma: immunopathology and prognosis. *Pathology*, **12**:3 (1980), 439–47.

17. Secco, G. B., Fardelli, R., Campora, E., *et al.* Primary mucinous adenocarcinomas and signet-ring cell carcinomas of colon and rectum. *Oncology*, **51**:1 (1994), 30–4.

18. Dukes, C. E. The classification of cancer of the rectum. *J Path Bact*, **35** (1932), 323.

19. Harrison, J. C., Dean, P. J., el-Zeky, F., and Vander Zwaag, R. From Dukes through Jass: pathological prognostic indicators in rectal cancer [see comments]. *Hum Pathol*, **25**:5 (1994), 498–505.

20. Jass, J. R. and Love, S. B. Prognostic value of direct spread in Dukes' C cases of rectal cancer. *Dis Colon Rectum*, **32**:6 (1989), 477–80.

21. Murano, A., Sasaki, F., Kido, C., *et al.* Endoscopic MRI using 3D-spoiled GRASS (SPGR) sequence for local staging of rectal carcinoma. *J Comput Assist Tomogr*, **19**:4 (1995), 586–91.

22. Joosten, F. B., Jansen, J. B., Joosten, H. J., and Rosenbusch, G. Staging of rectal carcinoma using MR double surface coil, MR endorectal coil, and intrarectal ultrasound: correlation with histopathologic findings. *J Comput Assist Tomogr*, **19**:5 (1995), 752–8.

23. Pegios, W., Vogl, J., Mack, M. G., *et al.* MRI diagnosis and staging of rectal carcinoma. *Abdom Imaging*, **21**:3 (1996), 211–18.

24. Vogl, T. J., Pegios, W., Mack, M. G., *et al.* Radiological modalities in the staging of colorectal tumors: new perspectives for increasing accuracy. *Recent Results Cancer Res*, **142** (1996), 103–20.

25. Okizuka, H., Sugimura, K., Yoshizako, T., Kaji, Y., and Wada, A. Rectal carcinoma: prospective comparison of conventional and gadopentetate dimeglumine enhanced fat-suppressed MR imaging. *J Magn Reson Imaging*, **6**:3 (1996), 465–71.

26. Willett, C. G., Badizadegan, K., Ancukiewicz, M., and Shellito, P. C. Prognostic factors in stage T3N0 rectal cancer: do all patients require postoperative pelvic irradiation and chemotherapy? *Dis Colon Rectum*, **42**:2 (1999), 167–73.

27. Cawthorn, S. J., Parums, D. V., Gibbs, N. M., *et al.* Extent of mesorectal spread and involvement of lateral resection margin as prognostic factors after surgery for rectal cancer [see comments]. *Lancet*, **335**:8697 (1990), 1055–9.

28. Merkel, S., Mansmann, U., Papadopoulos, T., *et al*. The prognostic inhomogeneity of colorectal carcinomas Stage III: a proposal for subdivision of Stage III. *Cancer*, **92**:11 (2001), 2754–9.

29. Brown, G., Radcliffe, A. G., Newcombe, R. G., *et al*. Preoperative assessment of prognostic factors in rectal cancer using high-resolution magnetic resonance imaging. *Br J Surg*, **90**:3 (2003), 355–64.

30. Brown, G., Richards, C. J., Newcombe, R. G., *et al*. Rectal carcinoma: thin-section MR imaging for staging in 28 patients. *Radiology*, **211**:1 (1999), 215–22.

31. Shepherd, N. A., Baxter, K. J., and Love, S. B. The prognostic importance of peritoneal involvement in colonic cancer: a prospective evaluation. *Gastroenterology*, **112**:4 (1997), 1096–102.

32. Shepherd, N. A., Baxter, K. J., and Love, S. B. Influence of local peritoneal involvement on pelvic recurrence and prognosis in rectal cancer. *J Clin Pathol*, **48**:9 (1995), 849–55.

33. Dukes, C. E., and Bussey, H. J. The spread of cancer and its effect on prognosis. *Cancer*, **12** (1958), 309–20.

34. Moran, M. R., James, E. C., Rothenberger, D. A., and Goldberg, S. M. Prognostic value of positive lymph nodes in rectal cancer. *Dis Colon Rectum*, **35**:6 (1992), 579–81.

35. Wolmark, N., Fisher, E. R., Wieand, H. S., and Fisher, B. The relationship of depth of penetration and tumor size to the number of positive nodes in Dukes C colorectal cancer. *Cancer*, **53**:12 (1984), 2707–12.

36. Andreola, S., Leo, E., Belli, F., *et al*. Manual dissection of adenocarcinoma of the lower third of the rectum specimens for detection of lymph node metastases smaller than 5 mm. *Cancer*, **77**:4 (1996), 607–12.

37. Chau, I., Allen, M., Cunningham, D., *et al*. Neoadjuvant systemic fluorouracil and mitomycin C prior to synchronous chemoradiation is an effective strategy in locally advanced rectal cancer. *Br J Cancer*, **88**:7 (2003), 1017–24.

38. Chau, I., Brown, G., Cunningham, D., *et al*. Neoadjuvant capecitabine and oxaliplatin followed by synchronous chemoradiation and total mesorectal excision in magnetic resonance imaging-defined poor-risk rectal cancer. *J Clin Oncol*, **24**:4 (2006), 668–74.

39. Adam, I. J., Mohamdee, M. O., Martin, I. G., *et al*. Role of circumferential margin involvement in the local recurrence of rectal cancer. *Lancet*, **344**:8924 (1994), 707–11.

40. Morita, T., Murata, A., Koyama, M., Totsuka, E., and Sasaki, M. Current status of autonomic nerve-preserving surgery for mid and lower rectal cancers: Japanese experience with lateral node dissection. *Dis Colon Rectum* **46**:suppl. 10 (2003), S78–87, discussion S87–8.

41. Suzuki, K., Muto, T., and Sawada, T. Prevention of local recurrence by extended lymphadenectomy for rectal cancer. *Surg Today*, **25**:9 (1995), 795–801.

42. Billingham, R. P. Extended lymphadenectomy for rectal cancer: cure vs quality of life. *Int Surg*, **79**:1 (1994), 11–22.

43. Moreira, L. F., Hizuta, A., Iwagaki, H., Tanaka, N., and Orita, K. Lateral lymph node dissection for rectal carcinoma below the peritoneal reflection. *Br J Surg*, **81**:2 (1994), 293–6.

44. Koch, M., Kienle, P., Antolovic, D., Buchler, M. W., and Weitz, J. Is the lateral lymph node compartment relevant? *Recent Results Cancer Res*, **165** (2005), 40–5.

45. Kikuchi, R., Takano, M., Takagi, K., *et al*. Management of early invasive colorectal cancer. Risk of recurrence and clinical guidelines [see comments]. *Dis Colon Rectum*, **38**:12 (1995), 1286–95.

46. Gall, F. P. Cancer of the rectum – local excision. *Int J Colorectal Dis*, **6**:2 (1991), 84–5.

47. Dworak, O. Morphology of lymph nodes in the resected rectum of patients with rectal carcinoma. *Pathol, Res Pract* **187**:8 (1991), 1020–4.

48. Hulsmans, F. H., Bosma, A., Mulder, P. J., Reeders, J. W., and Tytgat, G. N. Perirectal lymph nodes in rectal cancer: in vitro correlation of sonographic parameters and histopathologic findings. *Radiology*, **184**:2 (1992), 553–60.

49. Hildebrandt, U., Klein, T., Feifel, G., *et al*. Endosonography of pararectal lymph nodes. In vitro and in vivo evaluation. *Dis Colon Rectum*, **33**:10 (1990), 863–8.

50. Katsura, Y., Yamada, K., Ishizawa, T., Yoshinaka, H., and Shimazu, H. Endorectal ultrasonography for the assessment of wall invasion and lymph node metastasis in rectal cancer. *Dis Colon Rectum*, **35**:4 (1992), 362–8.

51. Brown, G., Richards, C. J., Bourne, M. W., *et al*. Morphologic predictors of lymph node status in rectal cancer with use of high-spatial-resolution MR imaging with histopathologic comparison. *Radiology*, **227**:2 (2003), 371–7.

52. Detry, R. J., Kartheuser, A. H., Lagneaux, G., and Rahier, J. Preoperative lymph node staging in rectal cancer: a difficult challenge. *Int J Colorectal Dis*, **11**:5 (1996), 217–21.

53. Spinelli, P., Schiavo, M., Meroni, E., *et al*. Results of EUS in detecting perirectal lymph node metastases of rectal cancer: the pathologist makes the difference. *Gastrointest Endosc*, **49**:6 (1999), 754–8.

54. Talbot, I. C., Ritchie, S., Leighton, M. H., *et al*. The clinical significance of invasion of veins by rectal cancer. *Br J Surg*, **67**:6 (1980), 439–42.

55. Horn, A., Dahl, O., and Morild, I. The role of venous and neural invasion on survival in rectal adenocarcinoma. *Dis Colon Rectum*, **33**:7 (1990), 598–601.

56. Horn, A., Dahl, O., and Morild, I. Venous and neural invasion as predictors of recurrence in rectal adenocarcinoma. *Dis Colon Rectum*, **34**:9 (1991), 798–804.

57. Heald, R. J. and Ryall, R. D. Recurrence and survival after total mesorectal excision for rectal cancer. *Lancet*, **1**:8496 (1986), 1479–82.

58. Bokey, E. L., Chapuis, P. H., Dent, O. F., *et al*. Factors affecting survival after excision of the rectum for cancer: a multivariate analysis. *Dis Colon Rectum*, **40**:1 (1997), 3–10.

59. Hall, N. R., Finan, P. J., al-Jaberi, T., *et al*. Circumferential margin involvement after mesorectal excision of rectal cancer with curative intent. Predictor of survival but not local recurrence? *Dis Colon Rectum*, **41**:8 (1998), 979–83.

60. Quirke, P. and Dixon, M. F. The prediction of local recurrence in rectal adenocarcinoma by histopathological examination. *Int J Colorectal Dis*, **3**:2 (1988), 127–31.

61. Quirke, P., Durdey, P., Dixon, M. F., and Williams, N. S. Local recurrence of rectal adenocarcinoma due to inadequate surgical resection. Histopathological study of lateral tumour spread and surgical excision. *Lancet*, **2**:8514 (1986), 996–9.

62. Sebag-Montefiore, D., Glynne-Jones, R., Mortensen, N., *et al.* Pooled analysis of outcome measures including the histopatological R0 resection rate after pre-operative chemoradiation for locally advanced rectal cancer. In Finan, P. J., ed., *Tripartite 2005 Colorectal Meeting* (Dublin, Ireland: Blackwell Publishing, 2005), p. 7.

63. Burton, S., Brown, G., Daniels, I., *et al.* MRI identified prognostic features of tumors in distal sigmoid, rectosigmoid, and upper rectum: Treatment with radiotherapy and chemotherapy. *Int J Radiat Oncol Biol Phys*, **65**:2 (2006), 445–51.

64. Bateman, A. C., Carr, N. J., and Warren, B. F. The retroperitoneal surface in distal caecal and proximal ascending colon carcinoma: the Cinderella surgical margin? *J Clin Pathol*, **58**:4 (2005), 426–8.

11

Imaging of metastatic disease

Gina Brown

Abstract

The case for intensive follow-up of patients with colorectal cancer has been strengthened in recent years by the success of treatment options for patients that develop metastatic disease. Nowhere is this strategy more cost-effective than in the early detection of isolated colorectal metastases since potentially curable recurrences will be detected by accurate imaging. Furthermore, utilizing FDG-PET with CT and MR scanning will lead to measurable benefits that supercede the costs incurred by such techniques.

At present, CT scanning of the thorax, abdomen, and pelvis remains the most useful modality for the surveillance of patients following colorectal surgery. Since the majority of patients develop metastatic disease within the first 2 years of surgery and it is relatively unusual to demonstrate metastatic disease after the first 5 years, it seems reasonable to intensify post-operative surveillance in the first 2 years with careful yearly CT follow-up assessment of patients at risk of developing metastatic disease thereafter. On occasion, the cause of a rising CEA level will not be demonstrated on conventional imaging. In these circumstances, FDG-PET is of value in identifying the focus of metastatic activity. Finally, FDG-PET provides a highly effective tool in further ensuring accurate selection of patients for resection by providing confirmation of the absence or presence of irresectable metastatic disease at other sites. Thus, the use of an accurate pre-operative screening technique that reliably selects patients using CT or MRI combined with FDG-PET will ensure appropriate patient selection for surgical resection.

Introduction

The early detection of metastatic disease in colorectal cancer either at initial presentation or during follow-up has been shown to benefit patients. This is because surgical resection for small volume isolated metastases can be curative and early detection of such disease improves the chances of cure. Even after metastatectomy, continued surveillance is worthwhile since repeat resection for recurrent disease is associated with favorable long-term survival [1,2,3]. Improvements in surgical technique mean that metastatectomy is also associated with very low post-operative morbidity ($<3\%$) so that increasingly surgery in patients over the age of 70 is successful with good outcomes. The task thus falls upon the multidisciplinary team to ensure that appropriate staging and follow-up strategies are in place to enable the detection of potentially resectable metastases. At the other end of the spectrum, patients with clearly inoperable metastatic disease at presentation should also be identified so that appropriate surgery or palliation can be planned. Surgical palliation with relatively short hospitalization is still an effective treatment since it alleviates many of the distressing symptoms that patients with metastatic colorectal disease suffer; improves survival compared with non-surgical supportive care; and patients benefit from palliative operations [4]. The percentage of patients in whom long-term cure is achievable following resection of metastatic disease in lungs or liver has increased in recent years and there is a continuing trend of improving survival and cure rates. Technological advances in imaging have played an important part in contributing to this improvement. This has been achieved through more accurate pre-operative imaging leading to rigorous patient selection [5,6,7].

Follow-up of patients with colorectal cancer

The relative merits of intensive image-based follow-up vs. a less intensive method have been subject to debate. The evidence base, however, appears to favor more intensive follow-up. For example, a meta-analysis suggested that more intensive follow-up combining CEA monitoring, outpatient clinical assessment, and yearly CT scanning improves survival compared with less intensive follow-up that does not utilize CT imaging [8]. The meta-analysis showed that intensive follow-up was associated with a reduced time to first relapse and significant absolute reduction in mortality rate of 9%–13%. Since these trials pre-dated the current wider trend of more aggressive hepatic resections and the use of combined therapies which, in their own right, have improved survival, it is likely that the potential survival benefit from intensive follow-up may be even greater than that identified in the meta-analysis. We evaluated 530 patients participating in a randomized, adjuvant chemotherapy clinical trial for stage II and III colon cancer who received CEA and CT scans of the chest, abdomen, and pelvis as a component of protocol-specific follow-up [9]. A nearly identical number of relapses were detected by CEA (45 relapses) and CT scan (49 relapses), and 14 were detected by both tests. Compared with those whose relapses were detected by symptoms (65 relapses), the CT-detected group had improved survival ($p = 0.0046$). Patients who were able to undergo potentially curative surgery had improved survival and were best detected by either CT scan (26.5%) or CEA (17.8%) compared with those with symptoms (3.1%, CT vs. symptomatic, $p < 0.001$; CEA vs. symptomatic, $p < 0.015$). As a result of this study and other meta-analyses, the American Society of Clinical Oncology has made the following recommendations:

- Annual computed tomography (CT) of the chest and abdomen for 3 years after primary therapy for patients who are at higher risk of recurrence and who could be candidates for curative-intent surgery;
- Pelvic CT scan for rectal cancer surveillance, especially for patients with several poor prognostic factors, including those who have not been treated with radiation;
- Colonoscopy at 3 years after operative treatment, and, if results are normal, every 5 years thereafter; flexible proctosigmoidoscopy every 6 months for 5 years for rectal cancer patients who have not been treated with pelvic radiation;
- History and physical examination every 3 to 6 months for the first 3 years, every 6 months during years 4 and 5, and subsequently at the discretion of the physician;
- Carcinoembryonic antigen every 3 months post-operatively for at least 3 years after diagnosis, if the patient is a candidate for surgery or systemic therapy;
- Chest X-rays, CBCs, and liver function tests are not recommended, and molecular or cellular markers should not influence the surveillance strategy based on available evidence.

In addition, the benefits of reviewing serial imaging in patients should not be neglected as it is an important method of increasing certainty of otherwise indeterminate lesions. For example, a lesion present and unchanged on both baseline and follow-up studies is unlikely to be malignant; on the other hand, a small malignant lung nodule is likely to double in size over 3 months.

Sites and mechanisms of metastatic disease in colorectal cancer

Hematogenous spread

Invasion of the extramural veins (Figure 11.1) is a known pre-disposing factor for the development of visceral metastatic disease, and its potential arises once colorectal cancer has invaded into the highly vascularized lamina propria. The

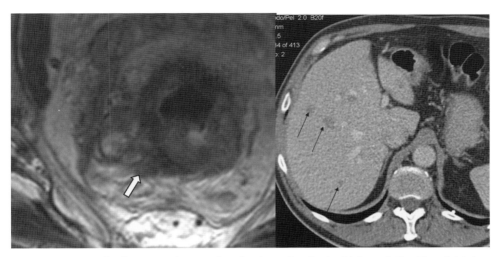

Figure 11.1 **Example of extramural venous invasion (arrow) on in vivo high-resolution T2-weighted axial image in a patient with rectal cancer, and synchronous metastases on CT (black arrows).**

link between extramural venous invasion and the subsequent development of metastatic disease is well established [10,11,12,13,14,15].

The liver is not only the most frequent site of metastatic disease but the sole site of metastasis in up to 30%–40% of colorectal patients. Metastatic disease to the lungs occurs in 15% of patients, ovarian metastases occurs in 6%–8% [16], bones metastases in 5%, and brain metastases in 5%. The spleen, kidneys, pancreas, adrenals, breast, thyroid, and skin are rarely involved. However, with the increased use of systemic agents and radiotherapy, these more unusual sites of metastatic disease are becoming more evident and appear to relate directly to the number of systemic therapies received [17].

Thoracic CT has been shown to improve the accuracy of pulmonary staging in colorectal cancer by allowing an appropriate treatment plan. Clearly, CT is likely to identify more benign radiological abnormalities than CXR alone. However, the baseline CT enables indeterminate lesions to be characterized more confidently on follow-up. In general, pulmonary metastases present as tiny nodules often less than 5 mm in diameter. The advent of multidetector CT enables much earlier detection of such lesions (Figure 11.2) and is therefore superior to any other modality in their detection [18].

Careful documentation of pulmonary metastases visualized on CT is worthwhile since the results of surgical lung resection show long-term survival advantage from both aggressive follow-up and surgery [19,20,21].

Ovarian metastases occur in 6%–8% of patients and may be easily mistaken for primary mucinous adenocarcinoma of the ovary (Figure 11.3) [16,22]. Several

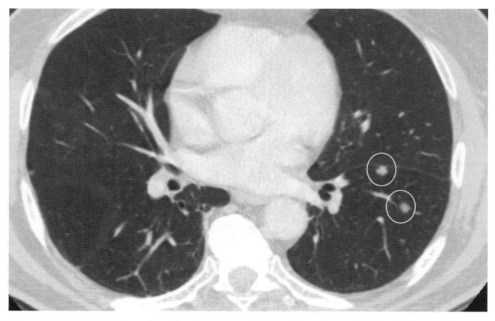

Figure 11.2 Early detection of small pulmonary metastatic disease in a patient on follow-up after curative resection of a colorectal primary tumor.

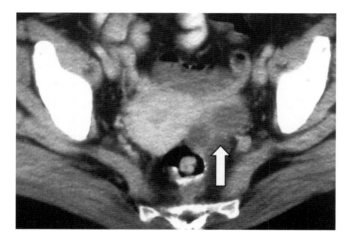

Figure 11.3 Ovarian metastatic disease presenting with primary colorectal carcinoma (arrow).

studies have described their CT appearances [22,23,24], namely large, lobulated or oval, multicystic or solid ovarian masses with a tendency for ovarian metastases to occur bilaterally [24].

The gross macroscopic and imaging findings may be identical to primary ovarian cancers and are only distinguished microscopically with difficulty by the presence of necrosis which suggests a colorectal origin. Much debate surrounds the usefulness of oophorectomy in such patients [25,26,27,28], and in the absence of a well-established evidence base, the decision to remove ovarian metastases surgically is made on an individual case basis [27].

Peritoneal metastases

The peritoneum is a relatively resistant barrier to spread but once a tumor has ulcerated through this layer, transcoelomic spread and intra-peritoneal deposits will ensue. Local peritoneal involvement is a common event in colorectal cancer and is an independent predictor of subsequent intra-peritoneal recurrence. It is known that such deposits have a pre-dilection for specific sites [29,30,31]:
- The superior and inferior ileocolic recesses
- The rectovesical pouch (Pouch of Douglas)
- The undersurface of the diaphragm
- The transverse mesocolon.

Poorly differentiated tumors are likely to produce diffuse seeding, whereas well-differentiated tumors are more likely to produce solitary deposits. Local peritoneal involvement is a common event in colon cancer and serves both as an important prognostic parameter as well as a consistent predictor of subsequent intra-peritoneal recurrence. Cases of metastatic peritoneal spread are most frequently because of perforation of the primary tumor through the peritoneal membrane. On occasion, this may be caused by intra-operative peritoneal spillage of malignant cells. Hydronephrosis can develop in patients with both right-sided and left-sided colonic primary tumors and in this group, tumor spread to the peritoneum, remote from the primary tumor site, is most often the cause of ureteric obstruction. The development of peritoneal deposits is mostly managed palliatively; however, in highly selected cases, good outcomes have been achieved surgically but require very careful workup and multimodality treatment (Figure 11.4) [32,33].

Lymph node spread

Lymph node metastasis is a progressive process with carcinoma spreading along lymphatic channels along anatomical pathways from node to node. In rectal cancers, this occurs as lateral spread to lymph nodes within the mesorectum, then laterally to locoregional nodes in the obturator fossa as well as upward spread along superior, middle and inferior rectal vessels, and internal iliac chain nodes (Figure 11.5). With left- and right-sided colonic primaries, nodal spread is along their draining

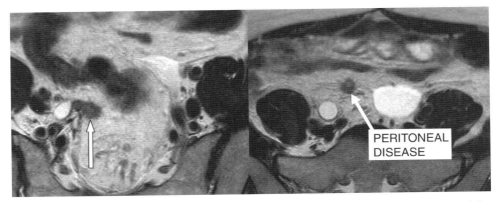

Figure 11.4 MRI images showing the typical appearance of peritoneal metastases (arrows) as nodular enhancing masses within the peritoneal cavity. Careful serial imaging review can be helpful in the early detection of subtle peritoneal disease and is a frequent cause of carcinoembryonic antigen elevation (tumor marker elevation).

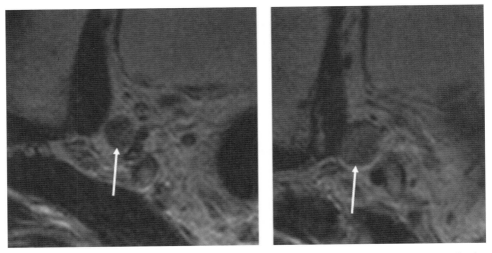

Figure 11.5 Axial MR image showing pelvic sidewall nodal disease as mixed signal intensity nodes in the internal iliac chain (arrow).

vessels, namely left colic artery and ileocolic vessels, respectively. When spread to the regional lymph nodes occurs, lymph flow can be blocked and so-called "retrograde" (downward) lymphatic metastasis may then occur. This is a rare occurrence in patients undergoing resection with curative intent; it is usually only apparent in advanced cancer and is associated with a poor prognosis. Spread to inguinal lymph nodes occurs rarely (approximately 2% of rectal cancers) and is usually associated with low rectal primaries growing into the anal canal.

Role of imaging in diagnosis and assessment of liver metastases

In selecting patients for curative hepatic resection, thin collimation CT or MR imaging of the liver with liver-specific contrast agents is of critical importance in delineating the distribution of metastases and assessing overall resectability. MR imaging has a further important role to play in characterizing co-existing benign lesions. The hepatic multidisciplinary team comprising the hepatobiliary surgeon, medical oncologist, radiologist and interventional radiologist, pathologist, and nurse specialist are essential in planning management of the patient since complex options for surgery and chemotherapy are required.

Increasingly, a wide range of imaging technologies and techniques are available and each performs differently in the pre-operative assessment of these patients. In practice, no one imaging modality will resolve all issues of patient selection and during review of cases in the multidisciplinary hepatic meeting the appropriate choice of complementing technologies enables rigorous patient selection and improved outcomes following hepatic resection for colorectal liver metastases. In pre-operative assessment of liver metastases, the following should be taken into account:

- Accurate delineation of anatomical distribution of metastases and segmental sparing in patients undergoing hepatic resection;
- Confirmation of absence of widespread multisegmental micrometastatic disease within the liver;
- Confirmation of absence of extrahepatic disease;
- Discrimination between coexisting benign lesions and metastases.

Prognostic factors governing outcomes after hepatic resection

The trend in improved survival following treatment for colorectal hepatic metastases may be attributed largely to improved techniques of anatomic resection [34,35,36], the availability of intra-operative ultrasonography [37,38], decreased mortality and morbidity in the peri-operative period [5], the use of second hepatic resections [39], and the use of chemotherapy [40,41,42,43]. The prognostic factors governing survival have been evaluated in a number of series but one of the largest was undertaken by Fong and colleagues based on experience of 1001 patients [44]. These have been recommended as a method of assigning a clinical risk score, with absence of any of these risk features conferring the highest survival advantage (60% 5-year survival) and 4 or more risk factors associated with poor (< 20% 5-year survival):

Clinical risk score

- Size > 5 cm
- Potential resection margin involved
- > 1 metastasis within liver
- Poor prognosis primary
- Synchronous primary/liver met < 12 months
- Extrahepatic disease.

All of these prognostic factors should be assessable by detailed pre-operative imaging which should enable rigorous patient selection; furthermore, intra-operative ultrasound has an important role in enabling precise localization and anatomic resection of lesions with tumor-free resection margins (Figure 11.6).

(A)

- Good prognostic score
  - Metachronous presentation (> 12 months)
  - Solitary metastasis
  - Low CEA
  - < 5 cm in diameter
  - Good prognosis primary

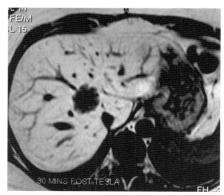

Figure 11.6   A) MR image of a good risk hepatic metastasis (arrow). The lesion is solitary, measures less than 4 cm in diameter, is not associated with an elevated carcinoembryonic antigen level, and the primary tumor was of a good prognosis. B) MR image of a poor risk hepatic metastatic disease; there is more than one lesion (arrows). Multiple lesions are shown and these measure more than 5 cm in diameter. The degree of segmental sparing is such that hepatic resection may result in potential resection margin involvement. Metastatic disease has been detected less than 12 months since primary surgery.

(B)

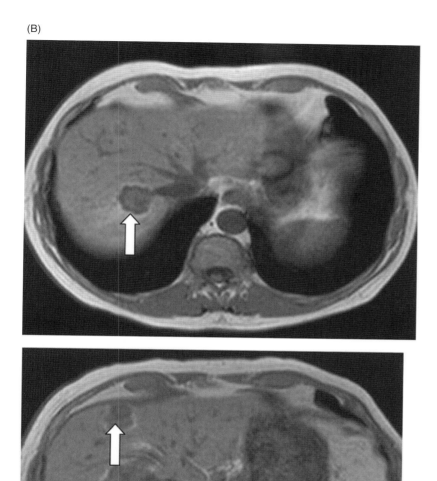

Figure 11.6   (cont)

Extrahepatic disease

It has been shown that patients with solitary unilobar tumors rarely have unrecognized irresectable disease, whereas patients with multiple bilobar tumors are at significantly higher risk of occult hepatic and extrahepatic disease [45]; these issues may influence the choice and intensity of pre-operative imaging investigations. The main tools for detecting coexisting extrahepatic disease are PET imaging, CT, and laparoscopy. Each is complementary, and it is important to recognize that each has its limitations and no single technique will identify all instances of extrahepatic disease.

Serial CT examinations of patients after colorectal cancer remain the most frequent follow-up imaging modality, and careful comparison of serial studies allows the distinction between benign non-malignant lesions in lung and liver. In many cases, the unequivocal demonstration of extrahepatic sites of disease by CT or multifocal irresectable liver disease will rule out hepatic surgery in the first instance. For the patients who appear potentially resectable following CT assessment, pre-operative FDG-PET has the greatest potential to alter outcomes by detection of extrahepatic disease not found on conventional imaging (Figure 11.7) [46]. By using FDG-PET imaging to select out patients with extrahepatic disease, unnecessary surgery was prevented in 6 out of 43 patients [46]. The precise anatomic location of intra-hepatic metastases was not always possible,

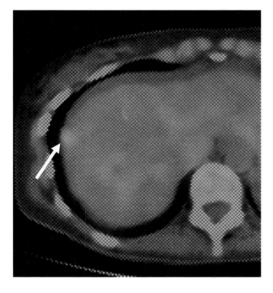

Figure 11.7   Example of PET-detected extrahepatic metastatic disease (arrow) in a patient with potentially resectable liver metastases.

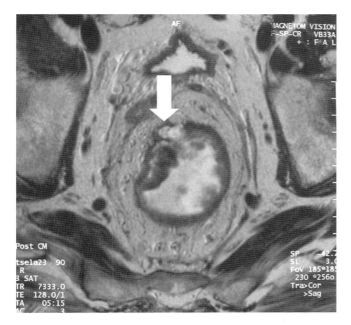

Figure 11.8 Example of disease relapse that was not FDG avid and therefore missed by 18-FDG PET CT (arrow).

however, using PET scanning. This may result in exclusion of such patients for resection. On the other hand, the demonstration of isolated extrahepatic disease by PET may result in multiple resections (e.g., lung metastatectomy and liver resection) that may potentially result in cure.

There are, however, some limitations of PET and CT imaging, particularly in their ability to identify small volume peritoneal disease (Figure 11.8) and surface disease on the liver.

In such patients, laparoscopy and intra-operative ultrasound may be the only methods of identifying these types of spread. Finally, there is evidence to suggest that the risk of extrahepatic disease is so low in patients with a clinical risk score of 0 that the use of 18FDG-PET in these circumstances is of limited value and has been shown to incorrectly upstage patients undergoing curative resection [47]. The authors suggested that 18FDG-PET should be reserved for those patients with a Fong clinical risk score of 1 or more.

The challenge that remains is the identification of disease that may be hard to detect by any imaging modality, namely small volume nodal metastases and peritoneal carcinomatosis, and failure to detect patients with these forms of spread will doubtless continue to contribute to instances of post-treatment failure. Future improvement in high-resolution imaging and lymph node-specific contrast agents may lead to enhanced patient selection.

Transabdominal ultrasound

Transabdominal ultrasound has not been proven to be as accurate as CT or MRI in the detection of liver metastases [48]. This is because assessment of such lesions is limited by the lack of inherent contrast between lesions and surrounding liver. Although ultrasound is less accurate at detecting metastases than CT, it is cheaper and more widely available and thus for some institutions may provide an effective screening or monitoring technique. However, it cannot be recommended in the pre-operative workup of patients considered for hepatic resection, as it is currently insufficiently accurate to predict resectability.

Ultrasound with contrast agents

In recent years, ultrasound microbubble contrast agents have gained in popularity and ease of use, and results show that the technique is at least equivalent to CT scanning in detection of lesions. It is particularly useful in the intra-operative setting, enabling tiny lesions to be visualized during hepatic resection or radio-frequency ablation procedures [49].

CT detection

Colorectal carcinomas metastasize to the liver by means of the portal venous system; however, they receive their blood supply from the hepatic artery [50]. CT, performed during peak level of hepatic parenchymal enhancement, will identify the vast majority of colorectal metastases and for many institutions, it is the modality of choice for the surveillance of patients at risk of developing liver metastases. The technique exploits the relative hypovascularity of colorectal neoplasms compared with normal parenchyma and results in accuracy rates of up to 85% (sensitivity 70%, specificity 94%) [51].

The improved sensitivity and specificity of helical CT reported by Valls [51] was attributed to thinner 5-mm collimation images compared with earlier CT studies employing slower scan times and 10-mm collimation. The issue of resectability has only been addressed in a few papers. In one series, 54% of patients thought to be resectable on pre-operative imaging were excluded by IOUS (intra-operative ultrasound) and laparoscopy. In another series, 78% were correctly identified as resectable representing a trend of improved pre-operative assessment which was improved further when a thin collimation technique was used. In this study, 94% of patients selected for hepatic resection by CT were found to be suitable for curative resection with a 58% 4-year survival rate [51]. Thus, higher spatial resolution CT techniques represent an improvement in the selection of patients suitable for curative hepatic resection.

Further improvements in CT technology with multidetector CT has largely negated the need for the more invasive CT-AP. Lesion detection at 10 mm or above is accurate and multidetector CT techniques achieve this improvement by virtue of its ability to achieve 1-mm isotropic voxel size with consequent improved spatial resolution and multiplanar capability [52].

These recent developments in multidetector scanners have enabled fast imaging of the entire liver within 10 seconds using new generation multidetector scanners and the potential to image during several phases of hepatic enhancement. However, although studies suggest that triple and biphasic techniques are of value in the assessment of hypervascular metastases, there is little convincing evidence for the value of arterial phase imaging in colorectal metastases [53,54]. Typically, colorectal hepatic metastases are demonstrated as hypodense lesions with rim enhancement (Figure 11.9). Larger lesions may contain central necrosis and thus contain a central low density "cystic" nidus.

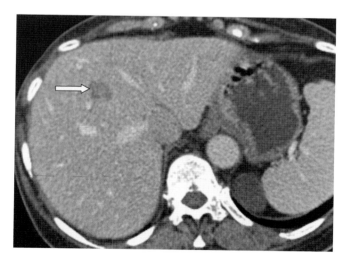

Figure 11.9   Typical appearance of hepatic metastases, visualized using multidetector CT (arrow).

Lesion characterization with CT

In addition to identification of liver metastases in patients with colorectal carcinoma, it is necessary to define an approach for distinguishing coincidental benign lesions that can potentially result in false-positive diagnosis.

Of these, cysts are the most commonly detected. Large lesions present little difficulty, as they are well defined, lack any rim enhancement, and have no internal architecture. Smaller lesions < 10 mm in diameter may be more difficult to characterize. The absence of any ring enhancement and the presence of a sharply delineated margin, and very low attenuation are helpful in distinguishing cysts from malignant lesions [55]. Arguably, MRI has superseded CT as the method of choice of characterizing potentially benign lesions.

Finally, the use of serial CT studies should not be neglected and is invaluable in determining the significance of lesions initially considered suspicious or indeterminate. The addition of a 3-month interval CT scan to compare with an initial assessment improves specificity from 0.91 to 0.99 [48].

MRI detection of liver metastases

MRI assessment

The workhorse of liver imaging is the T1-weighted gradient echo (GRE) sequence. It allows rapid imaging of the liver in a single breath-hold and can be acquired as a volume in axial or coronal planes enabling precise anatomic localization of lesions.

The recommended routines include a T1-weighted GRE. T2-weighted sequences will further aid characterization, and T1 in- and out-of-phase imaging are also rapid sequences which exploit the behavior of fat-containing tissues during in- and out-of-phase imaging. The sequence thus provides a useful means of further assessing apparent "perfusion defects" seen on CT which in some instances may be caused by focal fatty infiltration.

Gadolinium enhancement given as a rapid bolus can be achieved dynamically with images acquired in the arterial, portal venous, equilibrium, and delayed phases of enhancement. Semelka *et al.* [56] showed that MRI using dynamic contrast enhancement was superior to dual-phase spiral CT and was significantly superior for lesion characterization. It was further concluded that in terms of impact on patient management these differences had clinical significance. Thus, the ability of MRI to characterize structural abnormalities more reliably than CT is an advantage that can help in treatment planning and patient selection.

The increased sensitivity and specificity afforded by both superparamagnetic iron oxide (SPIO) and Mangafodipir as liver-specific agents has led to the more widespread use of MRI in the pre-operative assessment of patients with liver metastases. One of the first of such liver-specific agents to be evaluated was SPIO. Intra-venous infusion of this agent results in uptake by functioning Kupffer cells and darkening of the liver on MR imaging. Thus, metastases that do not contain Kupffer cells fail to take up this contrast and are shown up as relatively hyperintense lesions on SPIO-enhanced T1-weighted gradient echo images. However, other benign lesions can also show up as hyperdense, and care needs to be taken to ensure that false-positive lesions are not identified, particularly cysts and cavernous hemangiomas. Comparison with other sequences, especially the heavily T2-weighted sequence and the combined analysis of non-enhanced and SPIO sequences, is more accurate in the characterization of focal hepatic lesions than review of SPIO-enhanced images only [57]. MRI has shown considerable promise in overcoming the challenge of identifying lesions < 1 cm pre-operatively, and in a study evaluating the clinical impact of pre-operative assessment using SPIO compared with CT arterioportography (CTAP), it was shown that this technique was at least as accurate as spiral CTAP. Mangafodipir trisodium (Mn-DPDP) is taken up by the functioning hepatocytes and excreted by the biliary system. Contrast uptake leads to persistent elevation of T1-weighted signal of normal liver parenchyma within 10 minutes of injection. Comparison of T1-weighted images before and after administration of this agent shows a 100% increase in the signal to noise ratio of the liver and a 400% increase in conspicuity between the hypointense liver metastasis and surrounding parenchyma [58,59]. When compared with CT, the use of liver-specific agents increases the sensitivity and accuracy of detection of metastases. In a study comparing the performance of Mn-DPDP MRI with CT and intra-operative ultrasound, MRI influenced the operative decision in 74% [60]. Recent findings suggest that Mn-DPDP MRI is more sensitive than spiral contrast–enhanced CT in the pre-operative prediction of the resectability of hepatic lesions [60].

PET imaging

The diagnosis of tumors and metastatic disease using FDG-PET is based on increased regional glucose metabolism exhibited by tumor foci that is essentially independent of tumor size. In a meta-analysis comparing the performance of studies using ultrasound, CT, MR, and PET imaging in detection of gastrointestinal hepatic metastases, FDG-PET was the most sensitive imaging modality [61]. Furthermore, in a study by Park *et al.* [62], adopting a combined CT and FDG-PET was the most sensitive imaging modality and was found to be cost-effective for managing patients with elevated carcinoembryonic antigen levels who were candidates for hepatic resection.

Nonetheless, false-positive results can be obtained and this is a particular problem in patients that have received radiotherapy with false-positive results seen in the 6 months after radiotherapy caused by radiotherapy-induced granulation, fibroblast, and macrophage activity.

The technique may also yield false-positive results in detection of extrahepatic disease, particularly in granulomatous disease and inflammatory processes in the lung. Lesions < 1 cm in diameter may be a cause of false-negative diagnosis; micrometastatic disease in lymph nodes and the inability to separate nodes that lie in close proximity to the tumor are all limitations. It has therefore been suggested that in instances in which the findings of FDG-PET would result in the patient being denied potentially curative surgery then some other means of confirming the lesion is indicated. A careful attempt to localize and characterize a PET-detected abnormality should be sought by conventional imaging. Thus, the use of FDG-PET has transformed the way in which patients are selected for hepatic resection, but it is critical to provide anatomical details with conventional cross-sectional imaging for correct interpretation.

With improvements in outcome following surgery for the primary tumor, in particular the near virtual elimination of local recurrence, the challenge of detecting and treating metastatic disease becomes more important. We have a wide array of imaging modalities with which we can monitor patients, and the targeted and selective use of these modalities will enable better selection and appropriate treatments for recurrent disease.

REFERENCES

1. Petrowsky, H., Gonen, M., Jarnagin, W., *et al.* Second liver resections are safe and effective treatment for recurrent hepatic metastases from colorectal cancer: a bi-institutional analysis. *Ann Surg*, **235**:6 (2002), 863–71.
2. Shaw, I. M., Rees, M., Welsh, F. K., Bygrave, S., and John, T. G. Repeat hepatic resection for recurrent colorectal liver metastases is associated with favourable long-term survival. *Br J Surg*, **93**:4 (2006), 457–64.

3. Ogata, Y., Matono, K., Hayashi, A., *et al.* Repeat pulmonary resection for isolated recurrent lung metastases yields results comparable to those after first pulmonary resection in colorectal cancer. *World J Surg*, **29**:3 (2005), 363–8.

4. Cummins, E. R., Vick, K. D., and Poole, G. V. Incurable colorectal carcinoma: the role of surgical palliation. *Am Surg*, **70**:5 (2004), 433–7.

5. Choti, M. A., Sitzmann, J. V., Tiburi, M. F., *et al.* Trends in long-term survival following liver resection for hepatic colorectal metastases. *Ann Surg*, **235**:6 (2002), 759–66.

6. Wei, A. C., Greig, P. D., Grant, D., *et al.* Survival after hepatic resection for colorectal metastases: a 10-year experience. *Ann Surg Oncol*, **13**:5 (2006), 668–76.

7. Elias, D., Blot, F., El Otmany, A., *et al.* Curative treatment of peritoneal carcinomatosis arising from colorectal cancer by complete resection and intra-peritoneal chemotherapy. *Cancer*, **92**:1 (2001), 71–6.

8. Renehan, A. G., Egger, M., Saunders, M. P., and O'Dwyer, S. T. Impact on survival of intensive follow up after curative resection for colorectal cancer: systematic review and meta-analysis of randomised trials. *BMJ*, **324**:7341 (2002), 813.

9. Chau, I., Allen, M. J., Cunningham, D., *et al.* The value of routine serum carcino-embryonic antigen measurement and computed tomography in the surveillance of patients after adjuvant chemotherapy for colorectal cancer. *J Clin Oncol*, **22**:8 (2004), 1420–9.

10. Dukes, C. and Bussey, H. J. Venous spread in rectal cancer. *Proc R Soc Med*, **34** (1941), 571–3.

11. Sunderland, D. The significance of vein invasion by cancer of the rectum and sigmoid: a microscopic study of 210 cases. *Cancer*, **2** (1949), 429–37.

12. Lui, K. K., Enjoji, M., and Inokuchi, K. Venous permeation of colorectal carcinoma. *Jpn J Surg*, **10**:4 (1980), 284–9.

13. Talbot, I. C., Ritchie, S., Leighton, M. H., *et al.* The clinical significance of invasion of veins in cancer of the rectum. *Br J Surg*, **67**:6 (1980), 439–42.

14. Horn, A., Dahl, O., and Morild, I. Venous and neural invasion as predictors of recurrence in rectal adenocarcinoma. *Dis Colon Rectum*, **34**:9 (1991), 798–804.

15. Talbot, I. C., Ritchie, S., Leighton, M. H., *et al.* Spread of rectal cancer within veins. Histologic features and clinical significance. *Am J Surg*, **141**:1 (1981), 15–17.

16. Birnkrant, A., Sampson, J., and Sugarbaker, P. H. Ovarian metastasis from colorectal cancer. *Dis Colon Rectum*, **29**:11 (1986), 767–71.

17. Sundermeyer, M. L., Meropol, N. J., Rogatko, A., Wang, H., and Cohen, S. J. Changing patterns of bone and brain metastases in patients with colorectal cancer. *Clin Colorectal Cancer*, **5**:2 (2005), 108–13.

18. Reinhardt, M. J., Wiethoelter, N., Matthies, A., *et al.* PET recognition of pulmonary metastases on PET/CT imaging: impact of attenuation-corrected and non-attenuation-corrected PET images. *Eur J Nucl Med Mol Imaging*, **33**:2 (2006), 134–9.

19. Imdahl, A., Fischer, E., Tenckhof, C., *et al.* [Resection of combined or sequential lung and liver metastases of colorectal cancer: indication for everyone?]. *Zentralbl Chir*, **130**:6 (2005), 539–43.

20. McCormack, P. M., Burt, M. E., Bains, M. S., *et al.* Lung resection for colorectal metastases. 10-year results. *Arch Surg*, **127**:12 (1992), 1403–6.

21. Ike, H., Shimada, H., Ohki, S., *et al.* Results of aggressive resection of lung metastases from colorectal carcinoma detected by intensive follow-up. *Dis Colon Rectum*, **45**:4 (2002), 468–73, discussion 473–5.

22. Cho, K. C. and Gold, B. M. Computed tomography of Krukenberg tumors. *AJR Am J Roentgenol*, **145**:2 (1985), 285–8.

23. Kuhlman, J. E., Hruban, R. H., and Fishman, E. K. Krukenberg tumors: CT features and growth characteristics. *South Med J*, **82**:10 (1989), 1215–19.

24. Kim, S. H., Kim, W. H., Park, K. J., Lee, J. K., and Kim, J. S. CT and MR findings of Krukenberg tumors: comparison with primary ovarian tumors. *J Comput Assist Tomogr*, **20**:3 (1996), 393–8.

25. Perdomo, J. A., Hizuta, A., Iwagaki, H., *et al.* Ovarian metastasis in patients with colorectal carcinoma. *Acta Med Okayama*, **48**:1 (1994), 43–6.

26. Sielezneff, I., Salle, E., Antoine, K., *et al.* Simultaneous bilateral oophorectomy does not improve prognosis of post-menopausal women undergoing colorectal resection for cancer. *Dis Colon Rectum*, **40**:11 (1997), 1299–302.

27. Sakakura, C., Hagiwara, A., Yamazaki, J., *et al.* Management of post-operative follow-up and surgical treatment for Krukenberg tumor from colorectal cancers. *Hepatogastroenterology*, **51**:59 (2004), 1350–3.

28. Banerjee, S., Kapur, S., and Moran, B. J. The role of prophylactic oophorectomy in women undergoing surgery for colorectal cancer. *Colorectal Dis*, **7**:3 (2005), 214–17.

29. DeMeo, J. H., Fulcher, A. S., and Austin, R. F., Jr. Anatomic CT demonstration of the peritoneal spaces, ligaments, and mesenteries: normal and pathologic processes. *Radiographics*, **15**:4 (1995), 755–70.

30. Coakley, F. V. and Hricak, H. Imaging of peritoneal and mesenteric disease: key concepts for the clinical radiologist. *Clin Radiol*, **54**:9 (1999), 563–74.

31. Meyers, M. A., Oliphant, M., Berne, A. S., and Feldberg, M. A. The peritoneal ligaments and mesenteries: pathways of intra-abdominal spread of disease. *Radiology*, **163**:3 (1987), 593–604.

32. Glehen, O., Kwiatkowski, F., Sugarbaker, P. H., *et al.* Cytoreductive surgery combined with peri-operative intra-peritoneal chemotherapy for the management of peritoneal carcinomatosis from colorectal cancer: a multi-institutional study. *J Clin Oncol*, **22**:16 (2004), 3284–92.

33. Sugarbaker, P. H., Schellinx, M. E., Chang, D., Koslowe, P., and von Meyerfeldt, M. Peritoneal carcinomatosis from adenocarcinoma of the colon. *World J Surg*, **20**:5 (1996), 585–91, discussion 592.

34. Geoghegan, J. G. and Scheele, J. Treatment of colorectal liver metastases. *Br J Surg*, **86**:2 (1999), 158–69.

35. Jaeck, D., Bachellier, P., Guiguet, M., *et al.* Long-term survival following resection of colorectal hepatic metastases. Association Francaise de Chirurgie. *Br J Surg*, **84**:7 (1997), 977–80.

36. Fong, Y., Cohen, A. M., Fortner, J. G., *et al.* Liver resection for colorectal metastases. *J Clin Oncol*, **15**:3 (1997), 938–46.

37. Foroutani, A., Garland, A. M., Berber, E., *et al.* Laparoscopic ultrasound vs triphasic computed tomography for detecting liver tumors. *Arch Surg*, **135**:8 (2000), 933–8.

38. Cervone, A., Sardi, A., and Conaway, G. L. Intra-operative ultrasound (IOUS) is essential in the management of metastatic colorectal liver lesions. *Am Surg*, **66**:7 (2000), 611–15.

39. Nordlinger, B. and Wind, P. Repeat resections of primary hepatic malignancies. *Cancer Treat Res*, **69** (1994), 53–6.

40. Clavien, P. A., Selzner, N., Morse, M., Selzner, M., and Paulson, E. Downstaging of hepatocellular carcinoma and liver metastases from colorectal cancer by selective intra-arterial chemotherapy. *Surgery*, **131**:4 (2002), 433–42.

41. Shankar, A., Leonard, P., Renaut, A. J., *et al.* Neo-adjuvant therapy improves resectability rates for colorectal liver metastases. *Ann R Coll Surg Engl*, **83**:2 (2001), 85–8.

42. Adam, R., Avisar, E., Ariche, A., *et al.* Five-year survival following hepatic resection after neoadjuvant therapy for nonresectable colorectal. *Ann Surg Oncol*, **8**:4 (2001), 347–53.

43. Giacchetti, S., Itzhaki, M., Gruia, G., *et al.* Long-term survival of patients with unresectable colorectal cancer liver metastases following infusional chemotherapy with 5-fluorouracil, leucovorin, oxaliplatin and surgery. *Ann Oncol*, **10**:6 (1999), 663–9.

44. Fong, Y., Fortner, J., Sun, R. L., Brennan, M. F., and Blumgart, L. H. Clinical score for predicting recurrence after hepatic resection for metastatic colorectal cancer: analysis of 1001 consecutive cases. *Ann Surg*, **230**:3 (1999), 309–18, discussion 318–21.

45. Jarnagin, W. R., Fong, Y., Ky, A., *et al.* Liver resection for metastatic colorectal cancer: assessing the risk of occult irresectable disease. *J Am Coll Surg*, **188**:1 (1999), 33–42.

46. Strasberg, S. M., Dehdashti, F., Siegel, B. A., Drebin, J. A., and Linehan, D. Survival of patients evaluated by FDG-PET before hepatic resection for metastatic colorectal carcinoma: a prospective database study. *Ann Surg*, **233**:3 (2001), 293–9.

47. Schussler-Fiorenza, C. M., Mahvi, D. M., Niederhuber, J., Rikkers, L. F., and Weber, S. M. Clinical risk score correlates with yield of PET scan in patients with colorectal hepatic metastases. *J Gastrointest Surg*, **8**:2 (2004), 150–7, discussion 157–8.

48. Glover, C., Douse, P., Kane, P., *et al.* Accuracy of investigations for asymptomatic colorectal liver metastases. *Dis Colon Rectum*, **45**:4 (2002), 476–84.

49. Siosteen, A. K. and Elvin, A. Intra-operative uses of contrast-enhanced ultrasound. *Eur Radiol*, **14**:suppl. 8 (2004), P87–95.

50. Ridge, J. A., Bading, J. R., Gelbard, A. S., Benua, R. S., and Daly, J. M. Perfusion of colorectal hepatic metastases. Relative distribution of flow from the hepatic artery and portal vein. *Cancer*, **59**:9 (1987), 1547–53.

51. Valls, C., Andia, E., Sanchez, A., *et al.* Hepatic metastases from colorectal cancer: preoperative detection and assessment of resectability with helical CT. *Radiology*, **218**:1 (2001), 55–60.

52. Wong, K., Paulson, E. K., and Nelson, R. C. Breath-hold three-dimensional CT of the liver with multi-detector row helical CT. *Radiology*, **219**:1 (2001), 75–9.

53. Scott, D. J., Guthrie, J. A., Arnold, P., *et al.* Dual phase helical CT versus portal venous phase CT for the detection of colorectal liver metastases: correlation with intra-operative sonography, surgical and pathological findings. *Clin Radiol*, **56**:3 (2001), 235–42.

54. Ch'en, I. Y., Katz, D. S., Jeffrey, R. B., Jr., *et al.* Do arterial phase helical CT images improve detection or characterization of colorectal liver metastases? *J Comput Assist Tomogr*, **21**:3 (1997), 391–7.

55. Jang, H. J., Lim, H. K., Lee, W. J., *et al.* Small hypoattenuating lesions in the liver on single-phase helical CT in pre-operative patients with gastric and colorectal cancer: prevalence, significance, and differentiating features. *J Comput Assist Tomogr*, **26**:5 (2002), 718–24.

56. Semelka, R. C., Martin, D. R., Balci, C., and Lance, T. Focal liver lesions: comparison of dual-phase CT and multisequence multiplanar MR imaging including dynamic gadolinium enhancement. *J Magn Reson Imaging*, **13**:3 (2001), 397–401.

57. Reimer, P., Jahnke, N., Fiebich, M., *et al.* Hepatic lesion detection and characterization: value of nonenhanced MR imaging, superparamagnetic iron oxide-enhanced MR imaging, and spiral CT-ROC analysis. *Radiology*, **217**:1 (2000), 152–8.

58. Koh, D. M., Brown, G., Meer, Z., Norman, A. R., and Husband, J. E. Diagnostic accuracy of rim and segmental MRI enhancement of colorectal hepatic metastasis after administration of mangafodipir trisodium. *AJR Am J Roentgenol*, **188**:2 (2007), W154–61.

59. Young, S. W., Bradley, B., Muller, H. H., and Rubin, D. L. Detection of hepatic malignancies using Mn-DPDP (manganese dipyridoxal diphosphate) hepatobiliary MRI contrast agent. *Magn Reson Imaging*, **8**:3 (1990), 267–76.

60. Mann, G. N., Marx, H. F., Lai, L. L., and Wagman, L. D. Clinical and cost effectiveness of a new hepatocellular MRI contrast agent, mangafodipir trisodium, in the pre-operative assessment of liver resectability. *Ann Surg Oncol*, **8**:7 (2001), 573–9.

61. Kinkel, K., Lu, Y., Both, M., Warren, R. S., and Thoeni, R. F. Detection of hepatic metastases from cancers of the gastrointestinal tract by using noninvasive imaging methods (US, CT, MR imaging, PET): a meta-analysis. *Radiology*, **224**:3 (2002), 748–56.

62. Park, K. C., Schwimmer, J., Shepherd, J. E., *et al.* Decision analysis for the cost-effective management of recurrent colorectal cancer. *Ann Surg*, **233**:3 (2001), 310–19.

12

Patterns of recurrence following therapy for rectal cancer

Naureen Starling and Gina Brown

Introduction

The treatment of rectal cancer has evolved considerably over the last two decades from the employment of non-standardized surgery as the single modality of treatment to the development of standardized surgical techniques such as total mesorectal excision (TME) and the application of radiotherapy, chemoradiotherapy, and systemic chemotherapy either as single or combined modalities. Accompanying these developments have been improvements in local disease control and in some cases, survival from rectal cancer. Defining the rates and patterns of recurrence has been helpful in informing and developing each of these treatment strategies, local recurrence patterns indicating potential drawbacks of locally directed therapy and distant relapse indicative of the potential occult systemic component to the disease. Patterns and outcomes from recurrence have also helped to inform surveillance strategies, and here the recognition of recurrence, particularly within the pelvis, may be aided by standard categorization of local relapse patterns.

The impact of TME on local recurrence rates in rectal cancer

TME is defined as the resection of the rectum with its surrounding fatty and lymphatic tissue contained within the visceral sheet of the pelvic fascia. Pioneered by Heald in 1982, TME is a radical cancer operation based on the anatomy of fascial planes and fibrous spaces of the pelvis [1]. The technique was developed on the basis that residual tumor deposits are often seen circumferentially in the mesorectum distally from the lower edge of the rectal tumor and that resection of the entire mesorectum would therefore reduce the rate of local relapse [1,2,3]. The precise, sharp dissection of a TME proceeds in the nearly avascular

233

cleavage plane between the visceral and the parietal fascial sheets. This is in contrast to non-standardized, non-TME techniques that involve blunt dissection and which frequently result in tearing through the mesorectum.

Prior to the widespread adoption, in Europe at least, of TME for the treatment of rectal cancer, local recurrence (LR) rates of between 25% and 40% have been reported in large retrospective series of patients undergoing conventional, non-standardized surgery [4,5]. The Swedish Rectal Cancer Randomized Trial (SCRT), conducted between 1987 and 1990, was designed to evaluate conventional, non-standardized surgery with or without preoperative radiotherapy [6,7]. Of the 1168 patients randomized, 908 underwent curative surgery (R0; surgery with no evidence of gross or microscopic residual tumor) and within the surgery-alone arm ($n = 454$), an LR rate of 25% at 5 years was observed [7]. When all patients undergoing surgery were considered, including those deemed to have received non-radical surgery, the local recurrence rate was 27% at 5 years in the surgery-alone arm [6].

Since the introduction of TME, LR rates have fallen with reports in the literature of rates of between 4% and 11% in patients receiving surgery alone [3,4,8,9,10]. Heald *et al.* reported a case series of 405 consecutive rectal cancer patients treated with TME in which the 5- and 10-year LR rates were 3% and 4%, respectively, representing some of the lowest recurrence rates seen in trials of TME in this disease [11]. Although no randomized trials have directly compared TME with conventional surgical approaches, the body of evidence indicates that TME improves local tumor control. In one population-based study, the 4-year actuarial LR rate was 8% after TME compared to 23% in historical controls [12]. Whilst non-randomized, the two retrospective series mentioned earlier suggested improved survival and LR rates associated with the use of TME compared to conventional surgery [4,5]. Furthermore, in a Dutch randomized trial of preoperative radiotherapy in 1861 patients with rectal cancer who underwent TME according to stringent quality control measures [13], 2-year LR rates of 8.2% were documented in the surgery-alone arm ($n = 875$) compared to 16% in historical controls from an earlier study of conventional surgery alone [14]. In a comparison of these two trials, surgical technique (TME vs. non-TME) was found to be an independent prognostic predictor of local recurrence ($p = 0.002$) [15]. With longer follow-up, the LR in the surgery-only arm of the Dutch Rectal Cancer Trial was recently reported to be 11.3% at 5 years [16].

In the large series of TME performed in rectal cancer patients reported by Heald *et al.*, cancer-specific survival of all surgically treated patients was 68% at 5 years and 66% at 10 years [11]. Similarly, the 5-year cancer-specific and overall survival rates were 75%–80% and 62%–75% respectively in a pooled analysis of standardized surgery compared to 52% and 42%–44% for non-standardized surgery [5]. The latter is consistent with the 48% 5-year overall survival rates observed for the conventional surgery-only arm in the Swedish Rectal Cancer Trial. Although cross-study comparisons are inherently flawed for a multitude of reasons, the improvement of local therapy with TME and reduction in local recurrence therein appear to translate into a survival advantage for rectal cancer patients.

Factors predictive of local recurrence

Despite the impact of TME on LRs and prognosis for patients with rectal cancer, there are still subgroups of patients at significant risk of recurrence. T and N stage are recognized as independent prognostic variables for disease-free survival [17]. Importantly, the involvement of the circumferential resection margin (CRM) with tumor $\leq$ 1–2 mm from the CRM or a threatened CRM is also a predictor of LR and survival [2,18,19]. When TME is applied to anterior resections (ARs) and abdomino-perineal resections (APRs), the frequency of CRM involvement and LR rate is higher with APRs with one study indicating an LR rate of 22.3% vs. 13.5% ($p = 0.002$) for APRs compared to ARs, respectively [20]. This is in keeping with similar observations that lower rectal tumors with an inferior margin $\leq$ 6 cm from the anal verge are associated with higher rates of recurrence postoperatively [21] and is likely to be a reflection of the limited space available to achieve a full clearance of the mesorectum at this level in the pelvis. The latter study also indicated the prognostic significance of tumor stage, serosal, and venous invasion [21]. Within our cancer network, rectal cancers are grouped into intermediate, moderately high, or high risk for relapse based on these various predictors of recurrence. In general factors that have been selected as predictors of recurrence include T3c (invasion into perirectal fat > 5 mm) or T4 disease, node positive disease, low rectal tumors < 6 cm from the anal verge, CRM threatened or involved, and extramural venous invasion. This approach has helped to shape interventional strategies and clinical trial design for patients treated within our institution. This together with the pivotal role of preoperative thin slice MRI in this risk stratification has been discussed in more detail elsewhere.

Classifying patterns of local recurrence

Historically, identifying patterns of relapse, both local and distant, in series of patients undergoing conventional surgery for rectal cancer has been highly informative for identifying risk factors for recurrence and in the subsequent development of therapies directed at reducing recurrence rates. During the era when conventional surgery was performed as the sole treatment modality, several series documented patterns of relapse following surgery [22,23,24,25,26,27]. The definition of local and even distant recurrence often varied between series. In general, the definition of LR is restricted to the true pelvis or to include the superior extent of the radiotherapy field when this is used as part of a pre- or postoperative locally directed strategy.

Categorization of patterns of recurrence within the pelvis itself has been highly variable with no universally employed system in use. Authors have often referred to recurrence at specific sites such as the anastomosis, perineum, pre-sacral space, "elsewhere in the pelvis," or anterior vs. central or posterior recurrence. In one series, it was noted that the most common site of pelvis recurrence was within the pre-sacral space following conventional surgery alone [24]. In many cases, categorization of pelvic recurrence is not undertaken. The potential value of a universally employed categorization of pelvic recurrence lies in the standardization of review of postoperative surveillance scans, which may facilitate the recognition and early detection of recurrent disease.

We conducted an evaluation of patterns of recurrence in patients undergoing adjuvant chemotherapy for colorectal cancer as part of the randomized SAFFA trial [28] through independent radiological review of postoperative scans that were mandated as part of the trial [29]. Of the 801 patients enrolled, 323 has rectal or rectosigmoid cancer; and of these, 151 patients had tumors below the peritoneal reflection. Of these 151 patients, 61 relapsed and the pattern of local vs. distant relapse is shown in Table 12.1. Based on previous observations of patterns of recurrence, a classification system was devised to categorize recurrence according to marginal recurrence around the tumor bed (Figure 12.1(a)), lymph node (internal and external iliac groups) (Figure 12.1(b)), pelvic peritoneal (Figure 12.1(c)), perineal (Figure 12.1(d)), anastomotic (Figure 12.1(e)) and krukenberg (to the ovary) (Figure 12.1(f)). The frequency of these in our series is

Table 12.1 Frequency of local and distant relapse in patients treated with adjuvant chemotherapy within the SAFFA trial

Site of relapse	No. of patients	Median survival (months)
Pelvic only	23 (37.7%)	25.5
Distant only	20 (32.8%)	24.8
Pelvic and distant	18 (29.5%)	21.7

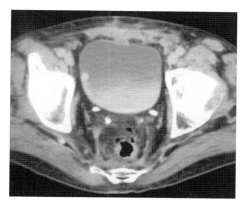 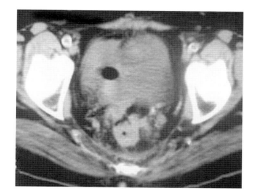

Figure 12.1(a)   Marginal.

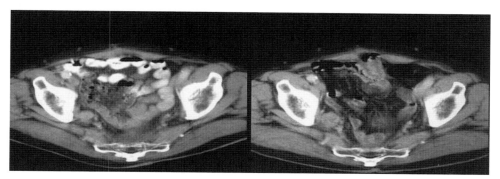

Figure 12.1(b)   Lymph node.

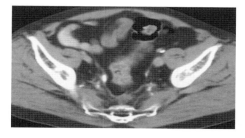 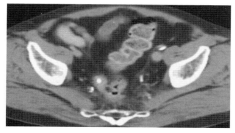

Figure 12.1(c)   Pelvic peritoneal.

indicated in Table 12.2. Marginal recurrence, as expected, was the most frequent pattern and given that the trial was undertaken before the widespread use of TME, we would expect the marginal pattern of recurrence to be significantly lower now. Perineal recurrence was most often seen when AP resections had been performed

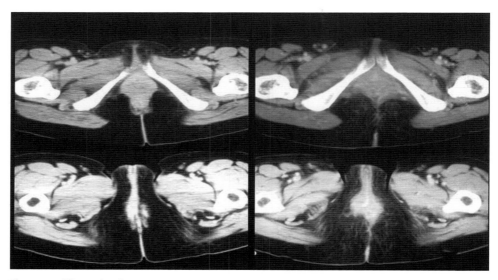

Figure 12.1(d)   Perineal.

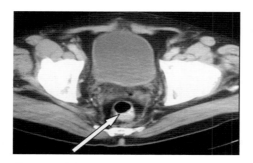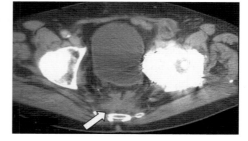

Figure 12.1(e)   Anastomotic.

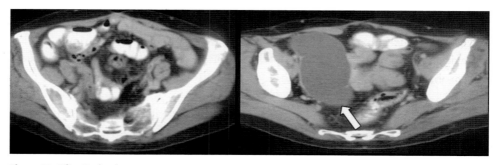

Figure 12.1(f)   Krukenberg.

Table 12.2 Frequency of patterns of local pelvic recurrence in patients treated with adjuvant chemotherapy within the SAFFA study

Relapse pattern	No. of patients, $n = 41$
(a) Marginal (around the margins of the surgical bed)	18/41 (43.9%)
(b) Lymph node (internal or external iliac groups)	10/41 (24.3%)
(c) Pelvic peritoneal[a]	9/41 (22.0%)
(d) Perineal	6/41 (14.6%)
(e) Anastomotic	5/41 (12.2%)
(f) Krukenberg	1/41 (2.4%)

[a] Peritoneal recurrence was associated with hydronephrosis in 7 of the 9 (78%) cases. This is likely to reflect the anatomical relations of the peritoneum and ureters. Hydronephrosis may be a marker of pelvic relapse.

and peritoneal recurrence was associated with hydronephrosis in the majority of cases (Figure 12.1(d)). The association of hydronephrosis with recurrent disease is recognized with some series noting an incidence of 7% to 19% in cases of recurrent rectal cancer [30,31,32]. All cases of recurrence could be classified using the suggested nomenclature. In particular, the marginal, perineal, and anastomotic patterns seem to represent failure of local surgical therapy.

Where pelvic CT is routinely undertaken as part of a surveillance program, which will be discussed later, or as part of a study mandated follow-up, the classification that we have suggested for rectal cancer recurrence may assist in the early recognition of recurrent disease. Comparison of current scans with the baseline postoperative scan is considered to be important in the recognition of recurrent disease, particularly in cases where recurrence is indolent and given that abnormalities on a postoperative scan that can be referred to as postoperative changes may actually represent residual/early recurrent disease. If suspicion exists regarding the latter, other imaging modalities such as PET, PET-CT, or MRI may have a role in helping to distinguish normal and tumor tissue but currently there is no evidence to support a routine clinical application. Resource utilization issues will probably restrict multimodality imaging to selected individual cases.

The impact of multimodality therapy on patterns of recurrence

A number of adjuncts have been applied to surgery, both pre- and post- the introduction of TME, in an attempt to improve LR rates and survival for rectal cancer. A comprehensive review of this field is beyond the scope of this book, hence key studies and their impact on recurrence rates have been selected.

In the USA, the standard of care is adjuvant chemoradiotherapy following rectal cancer surgery based on the results of the randomized trials of the Gastrointestinal Study Group (GITSG) and the North Central Cancer Treatment Group (NCCTG), neither of which utilized TME [33,34]. In the GITSG study, 202 patients were randomized between observation alone, chemotherapy, radiotherapy, or chemoradiotherapy followed by chemotherapy (combination therapy) [33]. The rate of LR was lower in the arms receiving any radiotherapy compared to those that did not (15/96 vs. 27/106) and with 94 months of follow-up, a 24% survival advantage was demonstrated for combination treatment compared to surgery alone [35]. In the NCCTG study, 204 patients were randomized between adjuvant radiotherapy or adjuvant combination chemoradiotherapy and chemotherapy [34]. With a median follow-up of over 7 years, the 5-year recurrence rate was 62.7% vs. 41.5% for the radiotherapy and combination treatments, respectively. LR as the first site of failure was lower in the combination arm (13.5% vs. 25.0%, $p = 0.036$) as was the rate of distant metastasis (28.8% vs. 46%, $p = 0.011$), and a survival advantage was demonstrated for the combination arm. A systemic approach to rectal cancer through the use of adjuvant chemotherapy is also supported by the results of the UK QUASAR study of adjuvant chemotherapy in colorectal cancer [36]; in the sub-group of patients with rectal cancer, adjuvant chemotherapy improved overall recurrence (19.6% vs. 26.8%, $p = 0.005$) and survival. The NSABP R-01 randomized trial of 555 patients failed to show a significant improvement in local control with postoperative radiotherapy [37]. However, a meta-analysis performed by the UK Colorectal Cancer Collaborative Group of 8 randomized trials including 2157 patients indicated that postoperative radiotherapy reduced the risk of isolated local recurrence at 5 years (15.3% vs. 22.9%, $p = 0.0002$) but not the risk of any recurrence (50.3% vs. 53.8%, $p = 0.10$) [38]. Survival was marginally better in those patients receiving any radiotherapy.

The role of preoperative radiotherapy either as a single modality or as part of a systemic combination approach to localized rectal cancer has also been extensively investigated in randomized studies and is considered the standard of care in several European centers. All of the trials utilizing single modality preoperative short course radiotherapy (25 Gy given in 5 fractions) [6,7,13,39,40] have demonstrated a significant improvement in LR rates in favor of preoperative radiation; in the Dutch TME trial, the 5-year LR was 11.4% vs. 5.8% ($p < 0.001$) and in the corresponding figures in the SRCT it was 27% vs. 11% (R0/R1, $p < 0.001$) [16].

The SRCT, however, was the only study to demonstrate a survival advantage for preoperative radiation. At median follow-up, 34% of patients in the curatively treated group had developed distant metastases with no significant differences on a stage-by-stage basis between the irradiated and surgery-alone groups, leading the authors to conclude that local control resulted in the survival gains observed [7]. Two meta-analyses have concluded that preoperative radiation significantly reduces the risk of LR [38,41], confers a survival benefit, and does not impact on the occurrence of distant metastases [41].

Chemoradiotherapy (CRT), that is the addition of chemotherapy as a radio-sensitizer to preoperative radiotherapy, has been evaluated in several randomized studies often with the aim of downstaging the primary and therefore frequently enrolling patients with unresectable or borderline resectable rectal cancers who are at increased risk of recurrent disease [42,43,44,45]. CRT is commonly based on 45 Gy to 54 Gy of pelvic radiation, including a boost to the tumor volume, administered over 5 to 6 weeks, and often utilizes fluoropyrimidine-based chemotherapy. Preoperative CRT appears to improve LR rates compared to radiotherapy alone but does not appear to impact on distant recurrence or indeed on survival [43,44].

In both pre- and postoperative strategies, the primary benefit of radiotherapy appears to be in improving local control, an effect that appears to be potentiated by the addition of a chemosensitizer. In general, radiotherapy with or without concurrent chemotherapy does not appear to influence the development of distant metastases. However, systemic approaches such as adjuvant chemotherapy either alone or sequential to pre- or postoperative CRT do appear to confer survival benefits, presumably through the treatment of occult micrometastatic disease. Analysis of the general patterns of recurrence, both local and distant, and survival parameters following these adjuncts to rectal cancer surgery have been instructive in the development of newer therapeutic strategies, many of which are incorporating systemic components to a multimodality treatment approach.

Follow-up after rectal cancer surgery for the detection of recurrence

The majority of LRs from rectal cancer occur within the first 2 years postoperatively [22,23,46]. LRs can be more indolent with reports of recurrences being identified up to 12 years post surgery [7]. In a series by Heald et al., almost all 5-year disease-free survivors were deemed cured following rectal cancer surgery, but in longer-term follow-up some late local and systemic recurrences were detected [47]. Given that radical approaches can be used in an attempt to cure certain cases of LR [48] and that isolated systemic recurrences can be amenable to resection with curative intent, there has been considerable interest in the value and nature of surveillance programs for colorectal cancer. Furthermore, LR is often a key endpoint of clinical studies evaluating therapies in rectal cancer whether it is defined simply as a rate or incorporated into disease or recurrence-free survival. It is therefore important that the patterns and outcomes of recurrence from rectal cancer are recognized and that recurrence is detected accurately and systematically.

The American Society of Clinical Oncology (ASCO) recently updated its *Practice Guidelines* for colorectal cancer surveillance [49]. Based on the evaluation of three meta-analyses of high and low-intensity surveillance programs [50,51,52] and several analyses of recent large trials in colorectal cancer, it was recommended that history and physical examination was undertaken every 3 to 6 months in the first 3 years, every 6 months in years 4 and 5 and thereafter at the discretion of the physician, and that the tumor marker CEA be taken every 3 months postoperatively for the first 3 years. CT scanning of the abdomen and chest was routinely recommended on an annual basis for the first 3 years. The addition of pelvic CT was recommended for rectal cancer surveillance in the presence of poor prognostic factors, and rectal proctosigmoidoscopy was recommended every 6 months for 5 years for patients who had not received pelvic radiation. In general, pelvic CTs were not mandated in the absence of poor prognostic features based on the observation in two studies that very few patients in whom local rectal recurrence was detected on the basis of a routine CT scan subsequently underwent curative resection [53,54]. One of the analyses informing this decision was performed at our institution [54]; as part of the SAFFA study described earlier [28,55], protocol-specific follow-up was mandated to include annual CT of the chest, abdomen, and pelvis annually for the first 2 years and routine history–examination and CEA 3-monthly for the first year, 6-monthly for the second year, and annually thereafter. The surveillance analysis also indicated that whilst the greater number of recurrences were abdominal, the larger proportion of resectable recurrences were thoracic. This together with the observation that pulmonary recurrences were as common as liver metastases and represented the largest proportion of resectable metastases in the INT 0114 rectal cancer study [56,57] led the panel to recommend routine thoracic CT as an addition to previous guidelines.

The recently published ESMO minimum guidelines for follow-up of rectal cancer [58] differ from the ASCO guidelines. History and rectosigmoidoscopy is recommended every 6 months for 2 years, and clinical, laboratory, and radiological examinations are considered to be of unproven benefit and recommended to be undertaken only in the presence of suspicious symptoms. However, at our institution, surveillance following rectal cancer surgery is similar to the guidelines set out by ASCO with slight variance; history-examination, and CEA are undertaken every 3 months for the first year, every 6 months for the second and third year, and annually for the fourth and fifth year. CT scanning of the chest and abdomen to include the pelvis is undertaken annually for 3 years and colonoscopic/sigmoidoscopic surveillance is also undertaken. As discussed earlier, classification of local pelvic relapse patterns according to standardized categorization may facilitate the recognition of local relapse during surveillance.

Conclusions

An understanding of the incidence, patterns, and associated outcomes of recurrence following therapy for rectal cancer has been instrumental in the development of both localized and systemic therapies for rectal cancer. The development of locally recurrent disease is largely a reflection of failure of the primary local therapy, whether this is surgery or radiotherapy, and analysis of local recurrence patterns has allowed the development and refinement of both these modalities. Strategies aimed at reducing local relapse are particularly important given the mortality and morbidity associated with pelvic recurrence and that once recurrence is detected, only a minority of cases can be cured. Standard categorization of local recurrence in the modern day may allow continued assessment of evolving locally directed therapies and facilitate the detection of recurrent disease. The latter may be particularly important when the rate of local recurrence is an endpoint of clinical studies of therapies in rectal cancer and in detection of recurrent disease in surveillance programs. Distant relapse is a reflection of the biological behavior of the disease and the presence of previously undetected micrometastatic disease. Hence analysis of the rates of distant relapse in rectal cancers has led to interest in the incorporation of systemic therapies to locally directed therapies, an approach reinforced by the observation of survival benefits seen with the administration of adjuvant chemotherapy. It is hoped that novel therapies and approaches to rectal cancer based on these patterns of recurrence and impact on survival will eventually further improve outcomes for patients with rectal cancer.

REFERENCES

1. Heald, R. J., Husband, E. M., and Ryall, R. D. The mesorectum in rectal cancer surgery – the clue to pelvic recurrence? *Br J Surg*, **69**:10 (1982), 613–16.

2. Quirke, P. and Dixon, M. F. The prediction of local recurrence in rectal adenocarcinoma by histopathological examination. *Int J Colorectal Dis*, **3**:2 (1988), 127–31.

3. Heald, R. J. and Ryall, R. D. Recurrence and survival after total mesorectal excision for rectal cancer. *Lancet*, **1**:8496 (1986), 1479–82.

4. Nesbakken, A., Nygaard, K., Westerheim, O., Mala, T., and Lunde, O. C. Local recurrence after mesorectal excision for rectal cancer. *Eur J Surg Oncol*, **28**:2 (2002), 126–34.

5. Havenga, K., Enker, W. E., Norstein, J., *et al.* Improved survival and local control after total mesorectal excision or D3 lymphadenectomy in the treatment of primary rectal cancer: an international analysis of 1411 patients. *Eur J Surg Oncol*, **25**:4 (1999), 368–74.

6. Improved survival with preoperative radiotherapy in resectable rectal cancer. Swedish rectal cancer trial. *N Engl J Med*, **336**:14 (1997), 980–7.

7. Folkesson, J., Birgisson, H., Pahlman, L., *et al.* Swedish rectal cancer trial: long lasting benefits from radiotherapy on survival and local recurrence rate. *J Clin Oncol*, **23**:24 (2005), 5644–50.

8. MacFarlane, J. K., Ryall, R. D., and Heald, R. J. Mesorectal excision for rectal cancer. *Lancet*, **341**:8843 (1993), 457–60.

9. Enker, W. E., Thaler, H. T., Cranor, M. L., and Polyak, T. Total mesorectal excision in the operative treatment of carcinoma of the rectum. *J Am Coll Surg*, **181**:4 (1995), 335–46.

10. Aitken, R. J. Mesorectal excision for rectal cancer. *Br J Surg*, **83**:2 (1996), 214–16.

11. Heald, R. J., Moran, B. J., Ryall, R. D., Sexton, R., and MacFarlane, J. K. Rectal cancer: the Basingstoke experience of total mesorectal excision, 1978–1997. *Arch Surg*, **133**:8 (1998), 894–9.

12. Arbman, G., Nilsson, E., Hallbook, O., and Sjodahl, R. Local recurrence following total mesorectal excision for rectal cancer. *Br J Surg*, **83**:3 (1996), 375–9.

13. Kapiteijn, E., Marijnen, C. A., Nagtegaal, I. D., *et al.* Preoperative radiotherapy combined with total mesorectal excision for resectable rectal cancer. *N Engl J Med*, **345**:9 (2001), 638–46.

14. Houbiers, J. G., Brand, A., van de Watering, L. M., *et al.* Randomised controlled trial comparing transfusion of leucocyte-depleted or buffy-coat-depleted blood in surgery for colorectal cancer. *Lancet*, **344**:8922 (1994), 573–8.

15. Kapiteijn, E., Putter, H., and van de Velde, C. J. Impact of the introduction and training of total mesorectal excision on recurrence and survival in rectal cancer in the Netherlands. *Br J Surg*, **89**:9 (2002), 1142–9.

16. Marijnen, C., Peeters, K., Putter, H., *et al.* Long term results, toxicity and quality of life in the TME trial. *Proc Am Soc Clin Oncol*, **23**: 16 Suppl. (2005).

17. Gunderson, L. L., Sargent, D. J., Tepper, J. E., *et al.* Impact of T and N stage and treatment on survival and relapse in adjuvant rectal cancer: a pooled analysis. *J Clin Oncol*, **22**:10 (2004), 1785–96.

18. Nagtegaal, I. D., Marijnen, C. A., Kranenbarg, E. K., van de Velde, C. J., and van Krieken, J. H. Circumferential margin involvement is still an important predictor of local recurrence in rectal carcinoma: not one millimeter but two millimeters is the limit. *Am J Surg Pathol*, **26**:3 (2002), 350–7.

19. Wibe, A., Rendedal, P. R., Svensson, E., *et al.* Prognostic significance of the circumferential resection margin following total mesorectal excision for rectal cancer. *Br J Surg*, **89**:3 (2002), 327–34.

20. Marr, R., Birbeck, K., Garvican, J., *et al.* The modern abdominoperineal excision: the next challenge after total mesorectal excision. *Ann Surg*, **242**:1 (2005), 74–82.

21. Tominaga, T., Sakabe, T., Koyama, Y., *et al.* Prognostic factors for patients with colon or rectal carcinoma treated with resection only. Five-year follow-up report. *Cancer*, **78**:3 (1996), 403–8.

22. Carlsson, U., Lasson, A., and Ekelund, G. Recurrence rates after curative surgery for rectal carcinoma, with special reference to their accuracy. *Dis Colon Rectum*, **30**:6 (1987), 431–4.

23. Rao, A. R., Kagan, A. R., Chan, P. M., *et al.* Patterns of recurrence following curative resection alone for adenocarcinoma of the rectum and sigmoid colon. *Cancer*, **48**:6 (1981), 1492–5.

24. Mendenhall, W. M., Million, R. R., and Pfaff, W. W. Patterns of recurrence in adenocarcinoma of the rectum and rectosigmoid treated with surgery alone: implications in treatment planning with adjuvant radiation therapy. *Int J Radiat Oncol Biol Phys*, **9**:7 (1983), 977–85.

25. Cass, A. W., Million, R. R., and Pfaff, W. W. Patterns of recurrence following surgery alone for adenocarcinoma of the colon and rectum. *Cancer*, **37**:6 (1976), 2861–5.

26. Pilipshen, S. J., Heilweil, M., Quan, S. H., Sternberg, S. S., and Enker, W. E. Patterns of pelvic recurrence following definitive resections of rectal cancer. *Cancer*, **53**:6 (1984), 1354–62.

27. Hruby, G., Barton, M., Miles, S., *et al.* Sites of local recurrence after surgery, with or without chemotherapy, for rectal cancer: implications for radiotherapy field design. *Int J Radiat Oncol Biol Phys*, **55**:1 (2003), 138–43.

28. Chau, I., Norman, A. R., Cunningham, D., *et al.* A randomised comparison between 6 months of bolus fluorouracil/leucovorin and 12 weeks of protracted venous infusion fluorouracil as adjuvant treatment in colorectal cancer. *Ann Oncol*, **16**:4 (2005), 549–57.

29. Starling, N., Brown, G., Tait, D., Norman, A., and Cunningham, D. Patterns of pelvic recurrence in patients with rectal cancers treated with adjuvant chemotherapy in a multicentre randomised study. *Proc Am Soc Clin Oncol*, **23**:16 suppl. (2005).

30. Larsen, S. G., Wiig, J. N., and Giercksky, K. E. Hydronephrosis as a prognostic factor in pelvic recurrence from rectal and colon carcinomas. *Am J Surg*, **190**:1 (2005), 55–60.

31. Cheng, C., Rodriguez-Bigas, M. A., and Petrelli, N. Is there a role for curative surgery for pelvic recurrence from rectal carcinoma in the presence of hydronephrosis? *Am J Surg*, **182**:3 (2001), 274–7.

32. Ulm, A. H. and Klein, E. Management of ureteral obstruction produced by recurrent cancer of the rectosigmoid colon. *Surg Gynecol Obstet*, **110** (1960), 413–18.

33. Prolongation of the disease-free interval in surgically treated rectal carcinoma. Gastrointestinal Tumor Study Group. *N Engl J Med*, **312**:23 (1985), 1465–72.

34. Krook, J. E., Moertel, C. G., Gunderson, L. L., *et al.* Effective surgical adjuvant therapy for high-risk rectal carcinoma. *N Engl J Med*, **324**:11 (1991), 709–15.

35. Douglass, H. O., Jr., Moertel, C. G., Mayer, R. J., *et al.* Survival after postoperative combination treatment of rectal cancer. *N Engl J Med*, **315**:20 (1986), 1294–5.

36. Gray, R. G., Barnwell, J., Hills, R., *et al.* QUASAR: a randomized study of adjuvant chemotherapy (CT) vs observation including 3238 colorectal cancer patients. *Proc Am Soc Clin Oncol*, **22**:14 suppl. (2004).

37. Fisher, B., Wolmark, N., Rockette, H., *et al.* Postoperative adjuvant chemotherapy or radiation therapy for rectal cancer: results from NSABP protocol R-01. *J Natl Cancer Inst*, **80**:1 (1988), 21–9.

38. Adjuvant radiotherapy for rectal cancer: a systematic overview of 8507 patients from 22 randomised trials. *Lancet*, **358**:9290 (2001), 1291–304.

39. Cedermark, B., Johansson, H., Rutqvist, L. E., and Wilking, N. The Stockholm I trial of preoperative short term radiotherapy in operable rectal carcinoma. A prospective randomized trial. Stockholm colorectal cancer study group. *Cancer*, **75**:9 (1995), 2269–75.

40. Martling, A., Holm, T., Johansson, H., Rutqvist, L. E., and Cedermark, B. The Stockholm II trial on preoperative radiotherapy in rectal carcinoma: long-term follow-up of a population-based study. *Cancer*, **92**:4 (2001), 896–902.

41. Camma, C., Giunta, M., Fiorica, F., *et al.* Preoperative radiotherapy for resectable rectal cancer: a meta-analysis. *JAMA*, **284**:8 (2000), 1008–15.

42. Sauer, R., Becker, H., Hohenberger, W., *et al.* Preoperative versus postoperative chemoradiotherapy for rectal cancer. *N Engl J Med*, **351**:17 (2004), 1731–40.

43. Bosset, J. F., Calais, G., Mineur, L., *et al.* Enhanced tumorocidal effect of chemotherapy with preoperative radiotherapy for rectal cancer: preliminary results – EORTC 22921. *J Clin Oncol*, **23**:24 (2005), 5620–7.

44. Bosset, J. F., Calais, G., Mineur, L., *et al.* Preoperative radiation (Preop RT) in rectal cancer: effect and timing of additional chemotherapy (CT) 5-year results of the EORTC 22921 trial. *Proc Am Soc Clin Oncol*, **23**:16 suppl. (2005).

45. Gerard, J., Bonnetain, F., Conroy, T., *et al.* Preoperative (preop) radiotherapy (RT) + 5 FU/folinic acid (FA) in T3–4 rectal cancers: results of the FFCD 9203 randomized trial. *Proc Am Soc Clin Oncol*, **23**:16 suppl. (2005).

46. Phillips, R. K., Hittinger, R., Blesovsky, L., Fry, J. S., and Fielding, L. P. Local recurrence following 'curative' surgery for large bowel cancer: I. The overall picture. *Br J Surg*, **71**:1 (1984), 12–16.

47. Moore, E., Heald, R. J., Cecil, T. D., *et al.* Almost all five year disease free survivors are cured following rectal cancer surgery, but longer term follow-up detects some late local and systemic recurrences. *Colorectal Dis*, **7**:4 (2005), 403–5.

48. Tepper, J. E., O'Connell, M., Hollis, D., *et al.* Analysis of surgical salvage after failure of primary therapy in rectal cancer: results from intergroup study 0114. *J Clin Oncol*, **21**:19 (2003), 3623–8.

49. Desch, C. E., Benson, A. B., III, Somerfield, M. R., *et al.* Colorectal cancer surveillance: 2005 update of an American Society of Clinical Oncology Practice Guideline. *J Clin Oncol*, **23**:33 (2005), 8512–19.

50. Figueredo, A., Rumble, R. B., Maroun, J., *et al.* Follow-up of patients with curatively resected colorectal cancer: a practice guideline. *BMC Cancer*, **3**: (2003), 26.

51. Renehan, A. G., Egger, M., Saunders, M. P., and O'Dwyer, S. T. Impact on survival of intensive follow up after curative resection for colorectal cancer: systematic review and meta-analysis of randomised trials. *BMJ*, **324**:7341 (2002), 813.

52. Jeffery, G. M., Hickey, B. E., and Hider, P. Follow-up strategies for patients treated for non-metastatic colorectal cancer. *Cochrane Database Syst Rev*, **1** (2002), CD002200.

53. Pietra, N., Sarli, L., Costi, R., *et al.* Role of follow-up in management of local recurrences of colorectal cancer: a prospective, randomized study. *Dis Colon Rectum*, **41**:9 (1998), 1127–33.

54. Chau, I., Allen, M. J., Cunningham, D., *et al.* The value of routine serum carcino-embryonic antigen measurement and computed tomography in the surveillance of patients after adjuvant chemotherapy for colorectal cancer. *J Clin Oncol*, **22**:8 (2004), 1420–9.

55. Saini, A., Norman, A. R., Cunningham, D., *et al.* Twelve weeks of protracted venous infusion of fluorouracil (5-FU) is as effective as 6 months of bolus 5-FU and folinic acid as adjuvant treatment in colorectal cancer. *Br J Cancer*, **88**:12 (2003), 1859–65.

56. Tepper, J. E., O'Connell, M. J., Petroni, G. R., *et al.* Adjuvant postoperative fluorouracil-modulated chemotherapy combined with pelvic radiation therapy for rectal cancer: initial results of intergroup 0114. *J Clin Oncol*, **15**:5 (1997), 2030–9.

57. Tepper, J. E., O'Connell, M., Niedzwiecki, D., *et al.* Adjuvant therapy in rectal cancer: analysis of stage, sex, and local control – final report of intergroup 0114. *J Clin Oncol*, **20**:7 (2002), 1744–50.

58. Tveit, K. M. and Kataja, V. V. ESMO minimum clinical recommendations for diagnosis, treatment and follow-up of rectal cancer. *Ann Oncol*, **1**: suppl. 16 (2005), i20–1.

Index